Images of Human Behavior

A Brain SPECT Atlas
Daniel G. Amen, MD

Brain Imaging Division

Amen Clinics, Inc.

Newport Beach, CA • Fairfield, CA • Tacoma, WA • Reston, VA

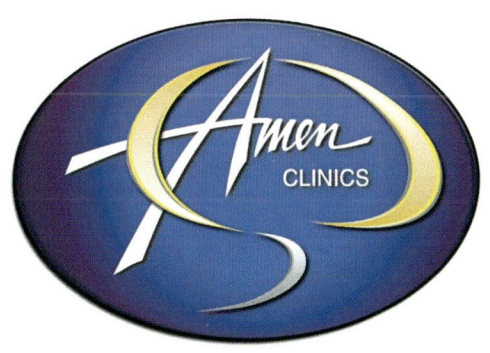

OTHER BOOKS BY DR. AMEN

HEALING A.D.D.
The Breakthrough Book That Allows You to See and Heal the 6 Types of A.D.D.

FIRESTORMS IN THE BRAIN
An Inside Look at Violent Behavior

CHANGE YOUR BRAIN, CHANGE YOUR LIFE
The Breakthrough Program for Conquering Anxiety, Depression, Obsessiveness, Anger and Impulsivity

HEALING THE HARDWARE OF THE SOUL
How Making the Brain-Soul Connection Can Optimize Your Life, Love, and Spiritual Growth

NEW SKILLS FOR FRAZZLED PARENTS
The Instruction Manual That Should Have Come With Your Child

MINDCOACH FOR KIDS
Teaching Kids and Teens to Think Positive and Feel Good

WOULD YOU GIVE TWO MINUTES A DAY FOR A LIFETIME OF LOVE?

TEN STEPS TO BUILDING VALUES WITHIN CHILDREN

A TEENAGER'S GUIDE TO A.D.D.

A CHILD'S GUIDE TO A.D.D.

PREVENTING ALZHEIMER'S
Ways to Help Prevent, Delay, Detect, and Even Halt Alzheimer's Disease and Other Forms of Memory Loss
With William Rodman Shankle, M.S., M.D.

HEALING ANXIETY AND DEPRESSION
With Lisa C. Routh, M.D.

SECRETS OF SUCCESSFUL STUDENTS
How to Be Your Best in School

TEACHER'S GUIDE TO ADD
Brain-Based Knowledge and Strategies for Helping ADD Students Succeed in School

ADD IN INTIMATE RELATIONSHIPS
A Comprehensive Guide for Couples

HOW TO GET OUT OF YOUR OWN WAY
A Step-by-Step Guide For Identifying and Achieving Your Goals

---

Confidentiality is essential to psychiatric practice. All case descriptions in this book, therefore, have been altered to preserve the anonymity of my patients without distorting the essentials of their stories.

The information offered in this book is not intended to be a substitute for the advice and counsel of your personal physician. Consult with your physician before making any medical changes.

Copyright 2004 by Daniel G. Amen, M.D.
All rights reserved. No part of this book may be reproduced or transmitted in any form or by any means without the written permission of the author.

ISBN #1-886554-04-8

Mindworks Press
4019 Westerly Place, Suite 100
Newport Beach, CA 92660
(949) 266-3730 Fax (949) 266-3770

Manufactured in the United States of America
9 8 7 6 5 4 3 2

Table of Contents

- v   **Examples of Brain SPECT Images**
- 1   **Brain Spect Imaging**
    - 1:1   An Introduction
    - 1:3   What is SPECT
- 2   **Normal Images**
    - 2:1   How SPECT is Interpreted
    - 2:2   Normal 3D Brain SPECT Studies
- 3   **Functional Neuroanatomy**
    - 3:2   The Deep Limbic System
    - 3:3   The Basal Ganglia System
    - 3:4   The Prefrontal Cortex
    - 3:5   The Anterior Cingulate Gyrus
    - 3:6   The Temporal Lobes
- 4   **Images of Strokes**
    - 4:1   Compelling Reasons Not To Smoke
    - 4:1   Left Frontal Stroke
    - 4:3   Two Right Sided Strokes
- 5   **Images of Dementia vs Psuedodementia**
    - 5:1   Alzheimer's Disease
    - 5:2   Pseudodementia
- 6   **Images of Brain Trauma**
    - 6:1   Wear a helmet, Avoid fights, No headers in soccer Wear your seatbelt, Play golf instead of football
    - 6:10   Fall from Roof
    - 6:11   24 Year Old Female Fall From Third Story
- 7   **Images of Depression**
- 8   **Images of Bipolar Disorder and Schizophrenia**
    - 8:1   Bipolar Disorder
    - 8:5   Schlzophrenla
- 9   **Images of the Ring of Fire**
    - 9:4   The Ring of Fire and Alcohol Induced Violence
- 10   **Images of Pms**
    - 10:1   Is it Real? You Bet!
    - 10:2   Haley
    - 10:4   Andrea
    - 10:6   Michelle
    - 10:7   JJ
    - 10:7   Chris
    - 10:10   Danielle

11   Images of Anxiety
      11:2   A Case of Post Traumatic Stress Disorder

12   Images of Attention Deficit Disorder
      12:1   Subtypes of ADD
      12:2   Rest, Concentration & Concentration wit Medication
      12:3   Before & After Treatment with Ritalin & Adderall

13   Images of Obsessive Compulsive Spectrum Disorders
      13:2   OCD
      13:3   ODD-Oppositional Defiant Disorder
      13:4   Road Rage
      13:5   Pathological Gambling
      13:6   Chronic Pain

14   Images of Violence
      14:2   John
      14:3   Bradley
      14:4   Rusty
      14:5   Jose
      14:6   Paul
      14:7   Steven
      14:8   Jody

15   Images of Alcohol and Drug Abuse
      15:1   Brain Pollution and the Real Reason You Shouldn't Use
      15:2   Marijuana
      15:3   Off and On Marijuana
      15:5   Heroin & Methadone
      15:6   Cocaine & Methamphetamine
      15:7   Alcohol
      15:9   Hope for Healing Alcohol, Cocaine & Meth

16   Images of Treatment
      16:1   Hope for Healing
      16:1   Paranoid Schizophreia
      16:3   Suicidal Rage
      16:4   Anger, ADD
      16:5   PTSD, Depression and Anxiety
      16:6   Attention Deficit Disorder
      16:8   Conduct Disorder
      16:9   Memory, Anger, ADD
      16:10 Asperger's Syndrome
      16:11 Severe Head Trauma
      16:12 Anger/Severe ODD

Examples of Brain SPECT Images

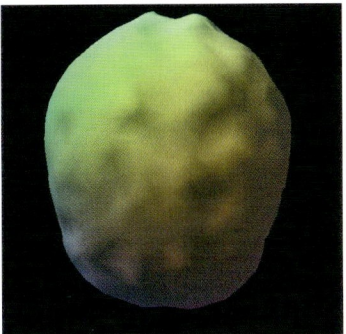

healthy top down surface view

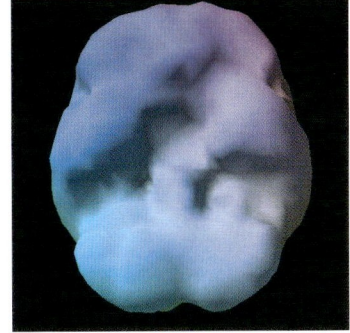

healthy bottom up surface view

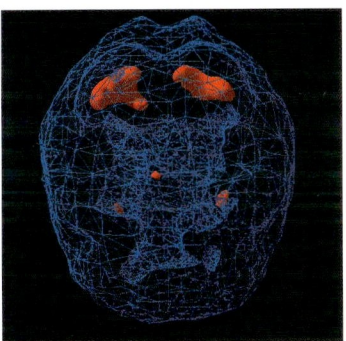

healthy top down active view

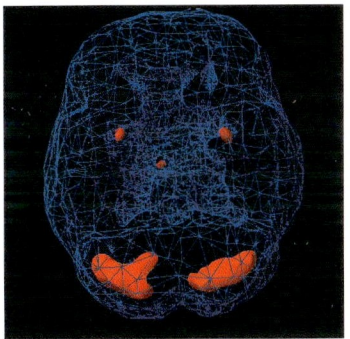

healthy bottom up active view

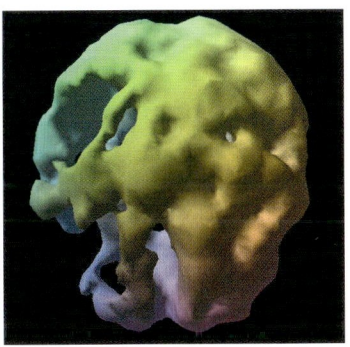

*top down surface view
2 right sided strokes*

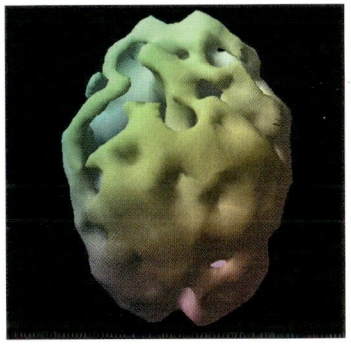

*top down surface view
Alzheimer's Disease*

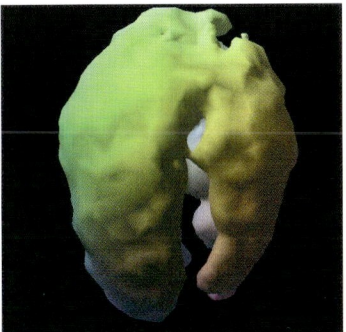

*top down surface view
brain trauma*

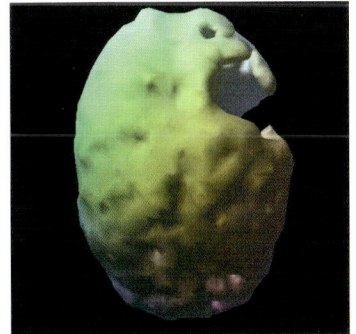

*top down surface view
brain trauma*

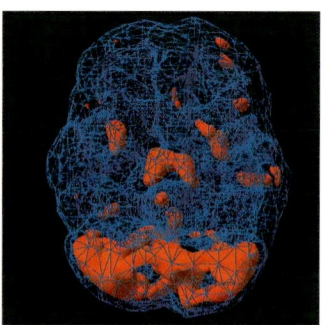

bottom up active view
depression
increased thalamo-limbic activity

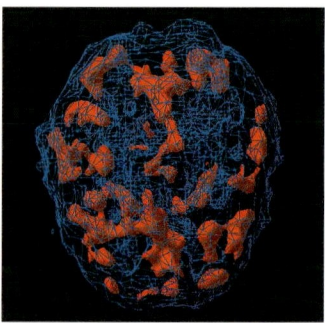

top down active view
bipolar disorder
patchy increased uptake

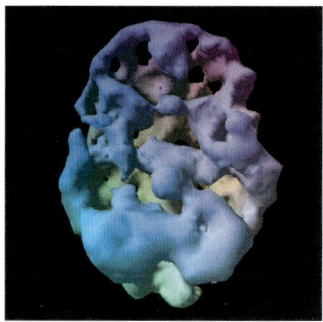

bottom up surface view
schizophrenia before treatment very
poor prefrontal activity

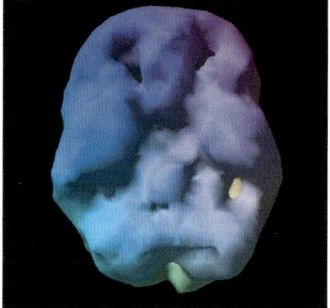

bottom up surface view
schizophrenia, after treatment with
Risperdal, improved overall activity

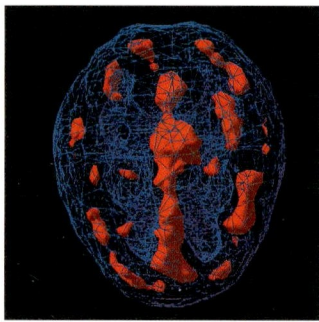

top down active view
obsessive compulsive disorder
marked increased cingulate activity

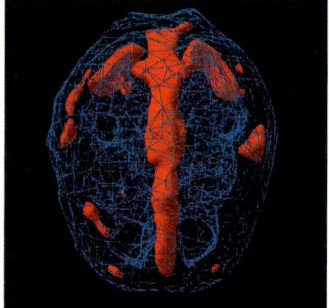

top down active view
oppositional defiant disorder
marked increased cingulate activity

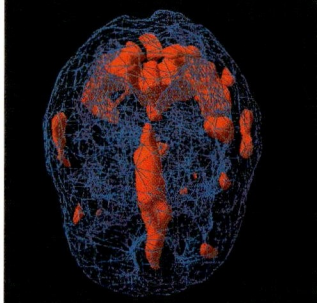

top down active view
PMS, during worst
time of cycle

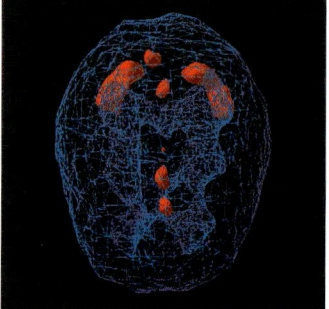

top down active view
PMS, during best time of cycle

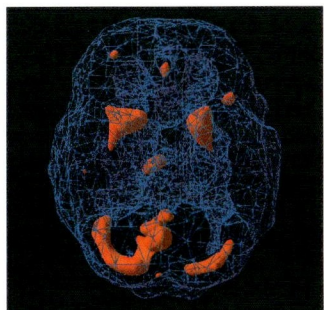

bottom up active view
generalized anxiety disorder
increased basal ganglia activity

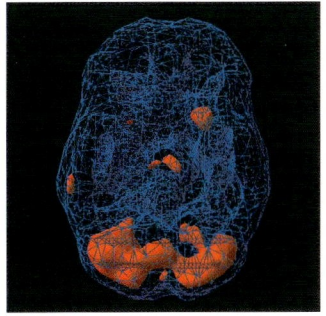

bottom up active view
panic disorder
increased left basal ganglia activity

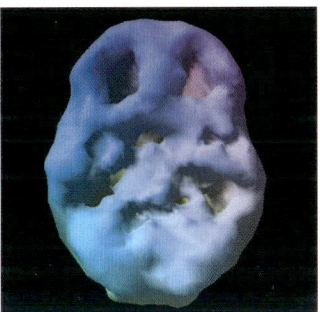

bottom up surface view
ADD, before treatment

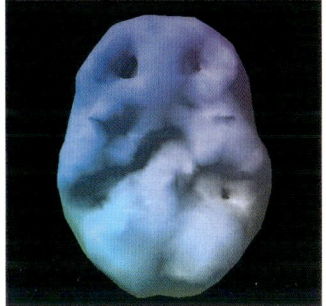

bottom up surface view
ADD, after treatment with Adderall

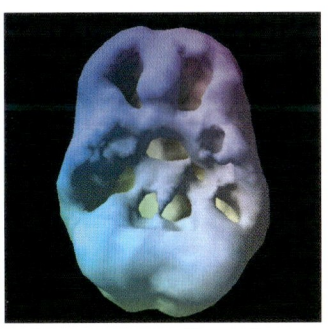

bottom up surface view
marijuana abuse, decreased
prefrontal and temporal lobe activity

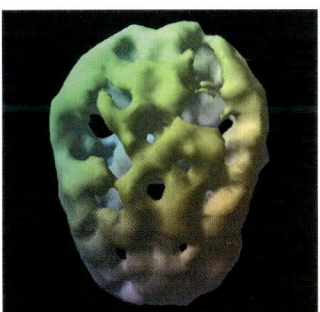

top down surface view
alcohol abuse
overall decreased activity

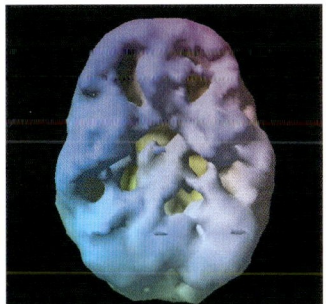

bottom up surface view
violent behavior,
before treatment

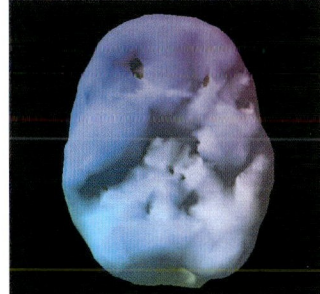

bottom up surface view
violent behavior, after treatment with
Neurontin and Adderall

Image Preparation: The SPECT surface images are rendered by setting the threshold at 55%, looking at the most active 45% of brain activity. The SPECT active images are rendered by setting the blue color threshold at 55%, looking at average brain activity in the brain, compared to the red threshold set at 85%, looking at the most active 15% of brain activity.

Section 1

Brain SPECT Imaging

An Introduction

On November 8, 1895 in Wurzburg Germany, Wilhelm Roentgen, a physicist at the University of Wurzburg, was working late in his laboratory. In an experiment he had been conducting before dinner, he had been sending an electric current through a tube. Without warning, a crystalline material on the other side of the room started emitting light. This made no sense to him. The rays produced by the tube could only travel a few centimeters; there was no way that they could travel all the way across the room to the crystal. Where was the light from the crystal coming from? When Roentgen came back after dinner, he tried the experiment again. This time he blackened the room, blocking out all light from the windows and covering the tube with black cardboard so no light could possibly escape when he sent another electric current through it. Still the crystalline material on the other side of the lab emitted visible light. Roentgen realized that it was caused by some kind of rays coming from the tube that were far more penetrating than he thought. Since he had never seen this phenomenon reported in the literature before and didn't know what the emitted rays were, he named them X-rays to signify their unknown nature.

Roentgen invited his wife Bertha into his lab to witness the experiment. The week before Christmas he made an X-ray of the bones in her left hand – the first X-ray ever of the human body.

After Roentgen published a short paper on the phenomenon, the newspapers sensationalized his discovery. The physicist's life was never the same again. In 1901 he won the first Nobel Prize in physics. An intensely private man, he did not relish the attention he got for his discovery. He certainly could not predict the impact his discovery would have on the lives of many millions of people.

Many remarkable inventions and discoveries came out of the second half of the 19th century in science, but it would be hard to overestimate the sensation Roentgen created with his skeletal photographs and the impact of his discovery on medicine, for it provided a way to see into the body without cutting it open. It was to be many years before scientists understood the true nature of X-rays. Roentgen did not, at the time, realize that what he had done was cause the crystal in his laboratory to emit visible radiation, when it was struck by X-rays from the vacuum tube. By bombarding the atoms of the crystal with the high energy photons from the X-rays, he had knocked the electrons of the crystal's atoms out of orbit. Whenever electrons move back from a higher energy orbit into a lower energy orbit they emit photons. This process is called electromagnetic radiation. Depending on where the emission is on the electromagnetic spectrum, it will be visible or not visible to the naked eye. In Roentgen's case, the electromagnetic rays were clearly visible.

Roentgen's first paper on the subject described about 40 different properties of his newly discovered X-rays. In 1896, another scientist, Henri Becquerel, read Roentgen's paper and noticed that these properties had a number of similarities to those he himself had observed in an unusual rock in his possession. When he first observed the rock, he did not realize it was emitting its own energy. He accidentally exposed some photographic plates to his uranium rock and he noticed changes consistent with Roentgen's discovery. But, where Roentgen had accidentally "created" radiation with his device, Becquerel was the first to discover the principal of naturally occurring radioactivity.

Marie Curie, one of Becquerel's students, found that certain samples of uranium had higher levels of activity than other samples. Upon investigation she discovered the reason: other elements, polonium (which gives off 700 times more radiation than uranium) and radium (which gives off a million times more radiation than uranium) were mixed in with the uranium ore. Radium and polonium were important in that they alerted scientists to the fact that there were particles in nature that produced their own energy, as opposed to everything else on Earth, which require energy from an outside source – the sun. For the next 40 years, other naturally occurring radioactive elements were discovered.

Radium was the first radioactive material ever used in medicine. However, it has an extremely long half-life (time it takes an isotope to decay from a level of radioactivity down to half that level). Simply for the sake of science, no one was interested in injecting a long-lived radioactive isotope into the body that was going to remain destroying cells for years to come. Therefore, when the medical possibilities for radioactive substances as a detection agent were recognized, scientists realized they needed to find an isotope that would do the job without doing any significant damage.

In Marie Curie's day, however, they were stuck with whatever nature had made available, and the radioactive materials occurring naturally had a half-life that lasted many, many years. It was important to scientists to be able to use radioactive substances with properties that allowed them to be safe inside the human body. In other words, they needed isotopes that would assist in understanding function and then disappear. Irene Curie (Marie's daughter) recognized this and found a way to artificially create radioactive material. Eventually technetium, was discovered and proved to be a very good short-acting isotope. It is the isotope we use in our lab. Of course, they could not possibly have known how to produce mass quantities of radioisotopes at the turn of the century. It was not until World War II, after the Manhattan Project developed the atomic bomb, that science was able to achieve that. The experimental nuclear reactor furnished a rich source of neutrons that generated radioisotopes in large quantities at a relatively low cost. From then on, there was no scarcity of radioactive material, for national defense or scientific research.

Many other important discoveries along the way helped nuclear medicine get where it is today. As early as 1903, Alexander Graham Bell suggested the first clinical use of radioactive material. In a letter he suggested the possibility that radium, in a sealed glass, tube could be inserted near a tumor in a patient. One of the most important discoveries, however, was made in 1927 in Boston by Herman Blumgart and his colleagues who used a diluted solution of radon to study circulation. By measuring how fast the diluted Radon flowed from one side of the body to the other, they were able to measure circulation and cardiac functions. Consequently they were the first to use radioactive isotopes to measure physiological functions in the body, and their discovery ushered in the "age of nuclear medicine." The studies of Dr. Blumgart and others conducted in the 1920s in observing the transportation of radioactive elements in the body lead to the conclusion that radioactive material could be used as a tracer. The "age of nuclear medicine" has created new and safer ways to treat people suffering from disease and injury.

What is SPECT?

What is SPECT? It is an acronym for Single Photon Emission Computerized Tomography. It is a sophisticated nuclear medicine study of cerebral blood flow and, indirectly, brain activity (metabolism).

A small amount of this compound is injected into the patient's vein where it runs through the blood stream and is taken up by certain receptor sites in the brain. The patient then lies on a table for 14-16 minutes while a SPECT "gamma" camera rotates slowly around his head. The camera has special crystals that detect where the compound (signaled by the radioisotope acting like a beacon of light) has gone. A supercomputer then reconstructs 3-D images of brain perfusion levels. The elegant brain snapshots that result offer a sophisticated blood flow/metabolism brain map. With these maps, physicians have been able to identify certain patterns of brain activity that correlate with psychiatric and neurological illnesses.

SPECT studies belong to a branch of medicine called nuclear medicine. Nuclear (refers to the nucleus of an unstable or radioactive atom) medicine uses radioactively tagged compounds (radiopharmaceuticals). The unstable atoms emit gamma rays when they decay, acting like a beacon of energy or light from each location. An unstable atom is always looking for stability, and will keep changing or degrading, until it reaches its most stable form. At each step of decay, it emits a gamma ray (portion of energy). Scientists can detect those gamma rays with film or special crystals and can record an accumulation of the number of beacons that have decayed in each area of the brain. These unstable atoms are essentially tracking devices – they track which cells were most active and had the most blood flow and those cells which are least active and have the least blood flow.

Nuclear medicine studies measure the physiological functioning of the body, and they can be used to diagnose a multitude of medical conditions: heart disease, certain forms of infection, the spread of cancer, and bone and thyroid disease. My own area of expertise in nuclear medicine, the brain, uses SPECT studies to help diagnose head trauma, dementia, atypical or unresponsive mood disorders, strokes, seizures, the impact of drug abuse on brain function and atypical or unresponsive aggressive behavior.

During the late 70s and 80s SPECT studies were being replaced, in many cases, by the sophisticated anatomical CT and later MRI studies. The resolution of those studies was far superior to SPECT as far as seeing tumors, cysts and blood clots. In fact, they nearly eliminated the use of SPECT studies altogether. Despite their clarity, CT scans and MRIs could only offer images of a static brain, and its anatomy; they gave little or no information on the activity in a working brain. It was analogous to looking at the parts of a car's engine without being able to turn it on. In the last decade it has become increasingly recognized that many neurological and psychiatric disorders are not disorders of the brain's anatomy, but problems in how it functions.

Two technological advancements have again encouraged the use of SPECT studies. Initially, the SPECT cameras were single-headed, and they took a long time to scan a person's brain (up to an hour). People had trouble holding still that long, and the images were fuzzy, hard to read (earning nuclear medicine the nickname "unclear medicine") and they did not give much information about the functioning deep within the brain. Then multi-headed cameras were developed, which were able to image the brain much faster and with enhanced resolution. The advancement of computer technology also allowed for improved data acquisition from the multi-headed systems. The brain SPECT studies of today, with their higher resolution, can see into the deeper areas of the brain with far greater clarity, and show what CT scans and MRIs cannot – how the brain actually functions.

Section 2

Normal Images

How SPECT is Interpreted

SPECT studies can be displayed in a variety of different ways. Traditionally, the brain is examined in three different planes: horizontally (cut from top to bottom), coronally (cut from front to back), and sagittally (cut from side to side). What do physicians see when they look at a SPECT study? They examine it for symmetry and activity levels indicated by shades of color (in different color scales selected depending on the physician's preference, including gray scales) and compare it to what they know a normal brain looks like. A normal SPECT image reveals homogeneous and uniform tracer accumulation throughout the cerebral cortex, with the cerebellum being the area of most intense perfusion. Chiron studied the normal progression of cerebral perfusion in children and found that by the age of 2 or 3 there is the same relative perfusion patterns as those seen in adults.

The images that accompany this atlas will be primarily two kinds of three dimensional (3D) images of the brain.

One kind is a 3D surface image, identifying the blood flow of the brain's cortical surface. These images are helpful in picking up cortical surface areas of good activity as well as underactive areas. They are helpful in examining strokes, brain trauma, the effects from drug abuse, etc. A normal 3D surface scan shows good, full, symmetrical activity across the brain's cortical surface.

The other kind is a 3D active brain image comparing average brain activity to the hottest 15% of activity. These images are helpful in picking up areas of overactivity, as seen in active seizures, obsessive compulsive disorder, anxiety problems, certain forms of depression, etc. A normal 3D active scan shows increased activity (seen by the red color) in the back of the brain (the cerebellum and visual or occipital cortex) and average activity everywhere else (shown by the background grid).

Physicians are usually alerted that something is wrong in one of three ways: (a) they see too much activity in a certain area; (b) they see too little activity in a certain area; or (c) they see asymmetrical areas of activity, which ought to be symmetrical

Normal 3D Brain SPECT Studies

back

top-down view

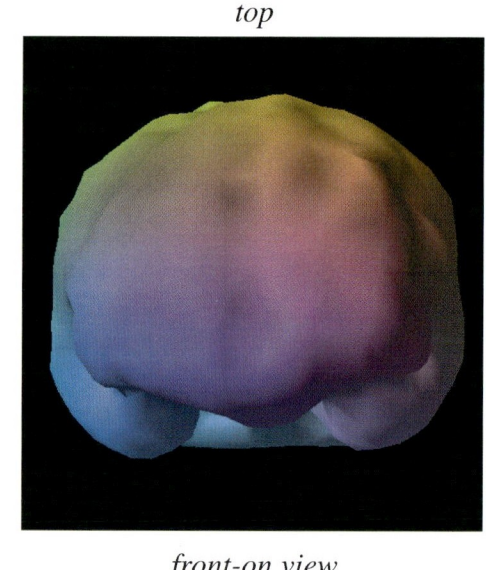

top

front-on view

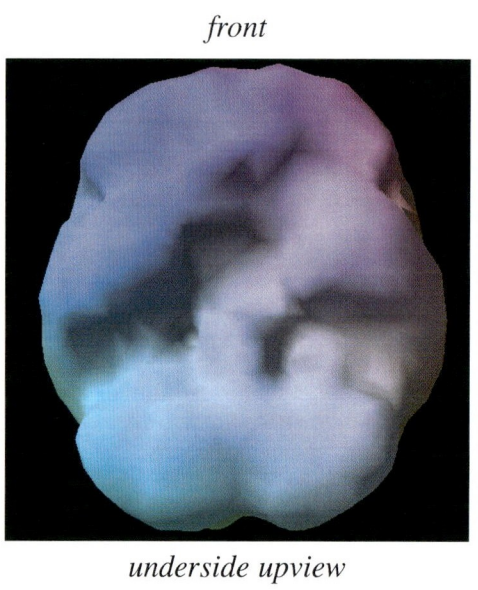

front

underside upview

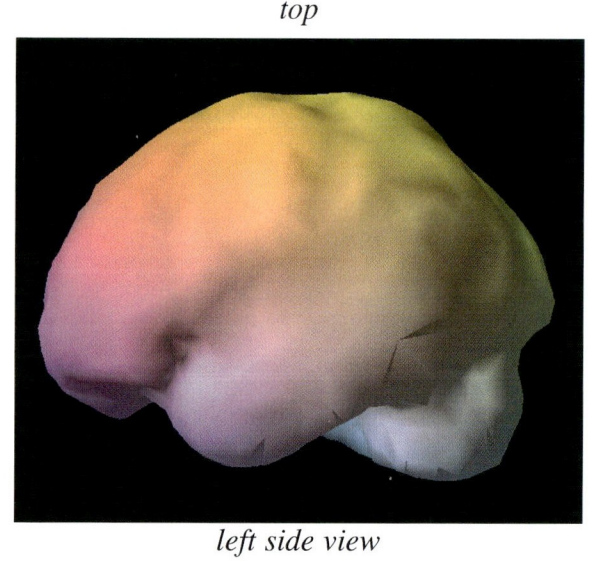

top

left side view

Normal Images

Normal 3D Brain SPECT Studies

back

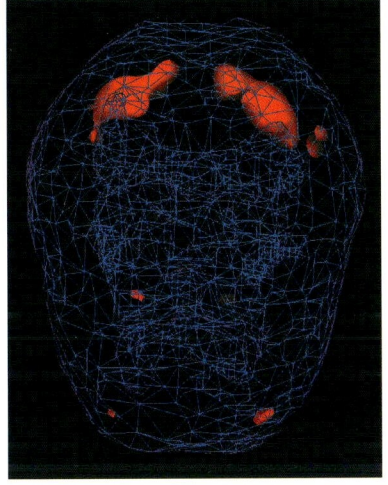

top-down view

top

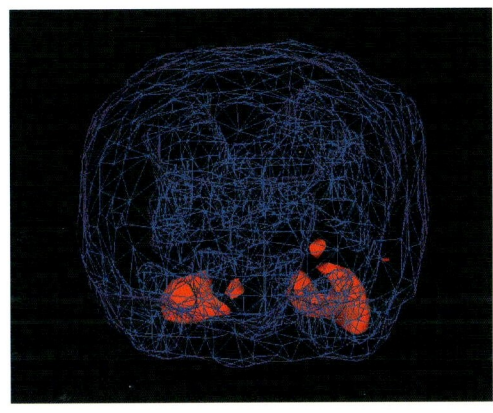

front-on view

front

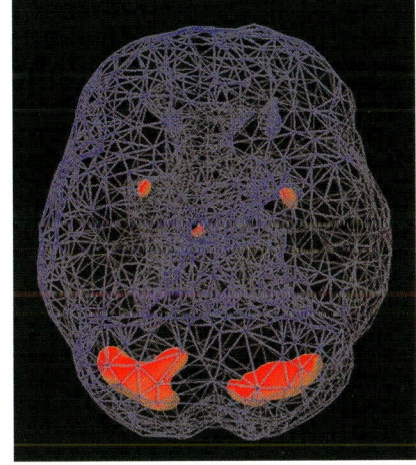

underside view

top

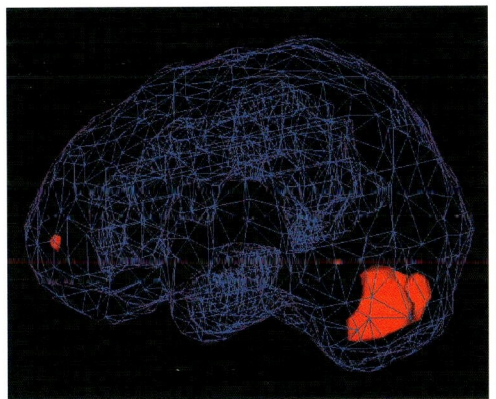

left side view

The surface images (1-4) are rendered by examining the most active 45% of brain activity. The active images are rendered by comparing the most active 45% or average brain activity (blue color) to the most active 15% (red or white color), the back of the brain is normally the most active part of the brain.

IMAGES OF HUMAN BEHAVIOR

SECTION 3

Functional Neuroanatomy

In order to understand this atlas, it is important to have a sense of the functional neuroanatomy of the brain. Over the next several pages there is a brief summary of the 5 major brain systems that relate to behavior, along with the general location of these areas seen on SPECT.

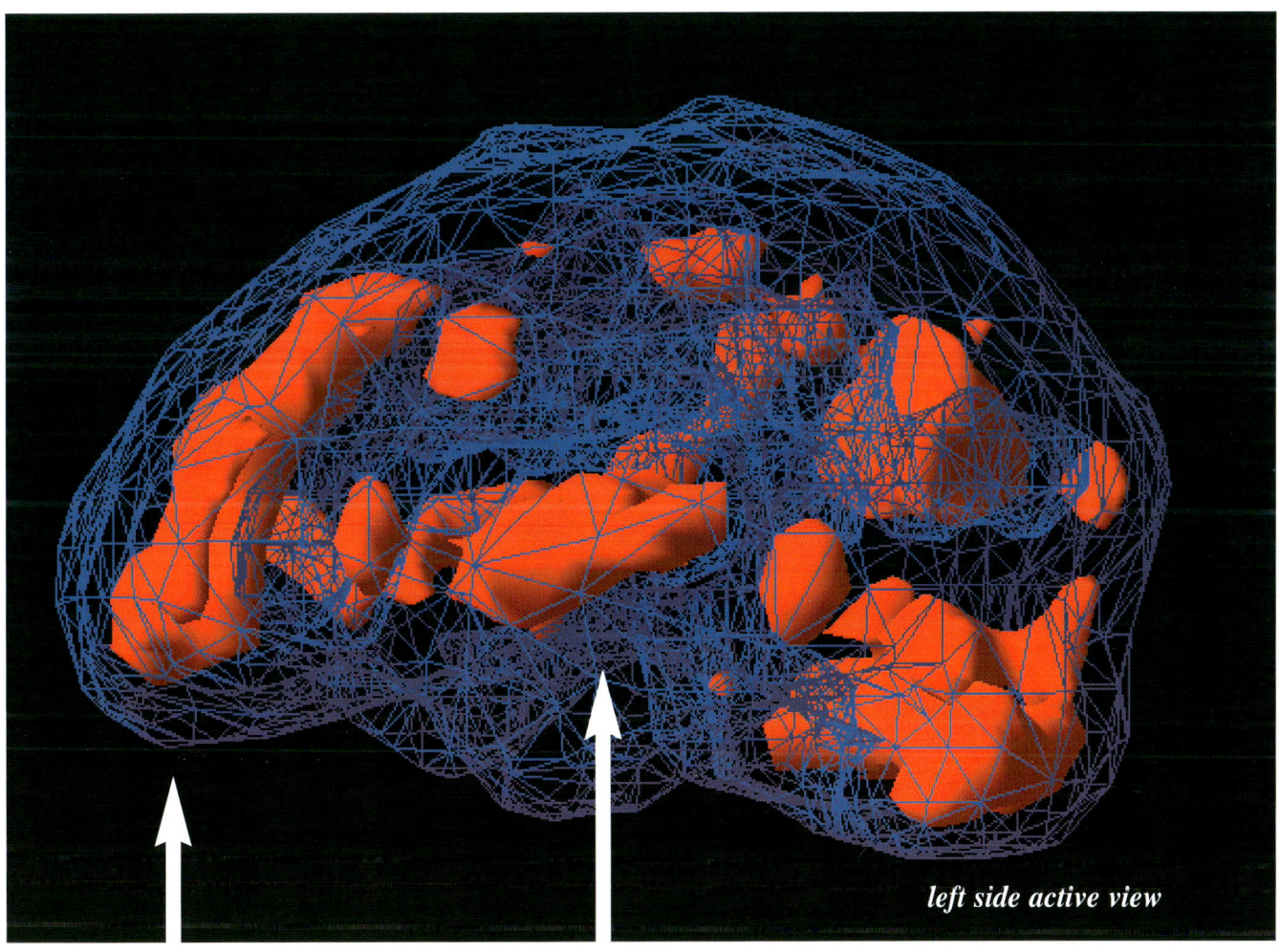

left side active view

anterior cingulate   *deep left temporal lobe*

The Deep Thalamo – Limbic System

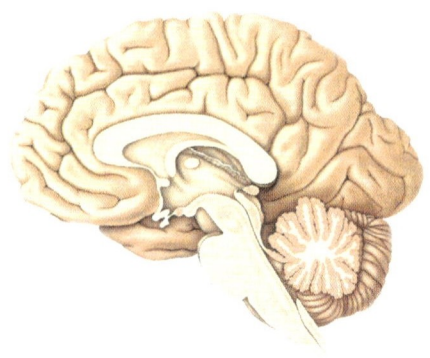
side view

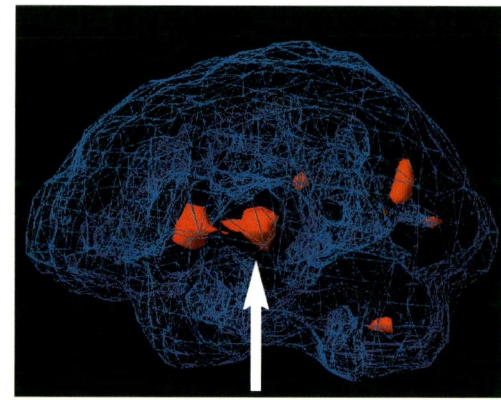
left side active view

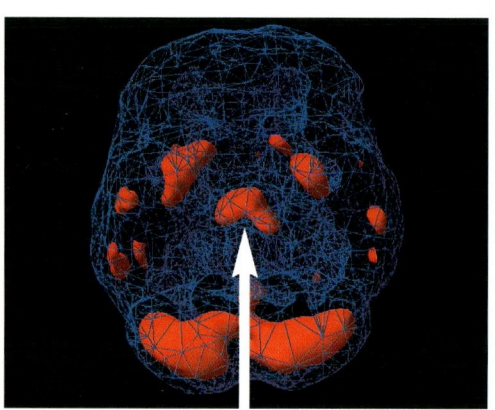
underside active view

Functions

- sets the emotional tone of the mind
- filters external events through internal states (emotional coloring)
- tags events as internally important
- stores highly charged emotional memories
- modulates motivation
- controls appetite and sleep cycles
- promotes bonding
- directly processes the sense of smell
- modulates libido

Problems

- moodiness, irritability, clinical depression
- increased negative thinking
- perceive events in a negative way
- decreased motivation
- flood of negative emotions
- appetite and sleep problems
- decreased or increased sexual responsiveness
- social isolation

The Basal Ganglia System

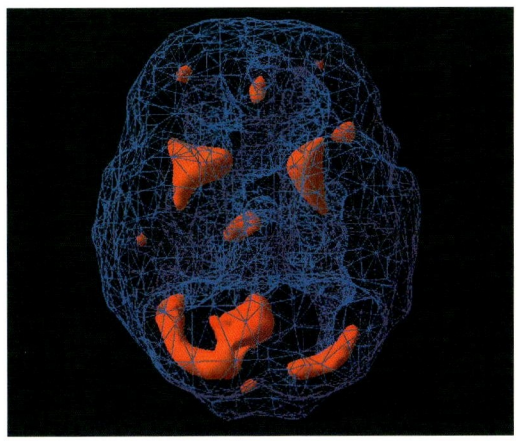

underside active view

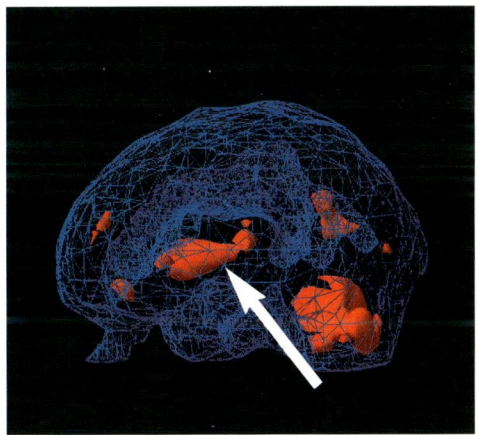

left side active view

Functions

- integrates feeling and movement
- shifts and smoothes fine motor behavior
- suppresses unwanted motor behaviors
- sets the body's idle or anxiety level
- enhances motivation
- pleasure/ecstasy

Problems

- anxiety, nervousness
- panic attacks
- physical sensations of anxiety
- tendency to predict the worst
- conflict avoidance
- Gilles de la Tourette's Syndrome/tics
- muscle tension, soreness
- tremors
- fine motor problems
- headaches
- low or excessive motivation

The Prefrontal Cortex

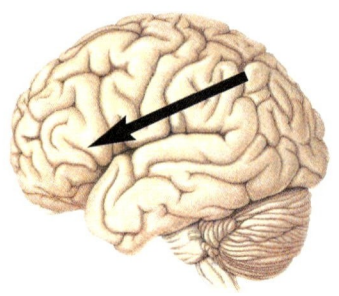

dorsal lateral prefrontal cortex outside view

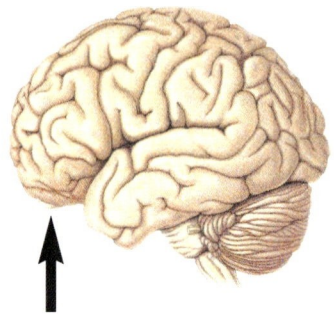

inferior orbital prefrontal cortex outside view

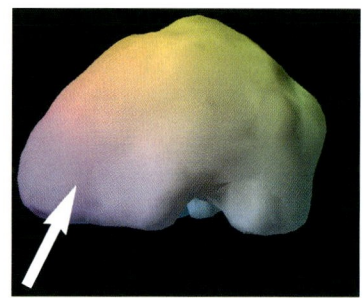

side surface view dorsal lateral prefrontal area

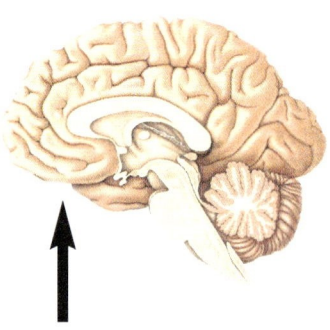

inferior orbital prefrontal area inside view

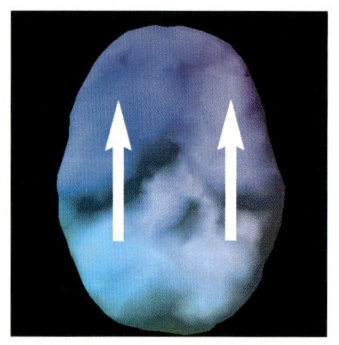

underside surface view inferior orbital prefrontal area

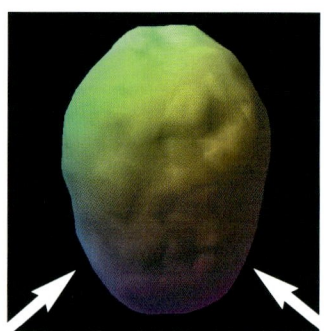

top-down surface view dorsal lateral prefrontal area

Prefrontal Cortex

Functions

- attention span
- perseverance
- judgment
- impulse control
- organization
- self-monitoring and supervision
- problem solving
- critical thinking
- forward thinking
- learning from experience
- ability to feel and express emotions
- influences the limbic system
- empathy

Problems

- short attention span
- distractibility
- lack of perseverance
- impulse control problems
- hyperactivity
- chronic tardiness, poor time management
- disorganization
- procrastination
- unavailability of emotions
- misperceptions
- poor judgement
- trouble learning from experience
- short term memory problems
- social and test anxiety

The Anterior Cingulate Gyrus

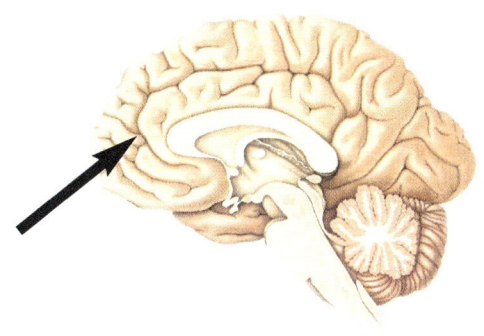
inside side view

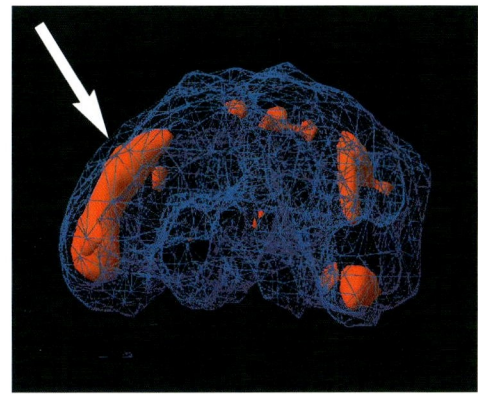
side active view

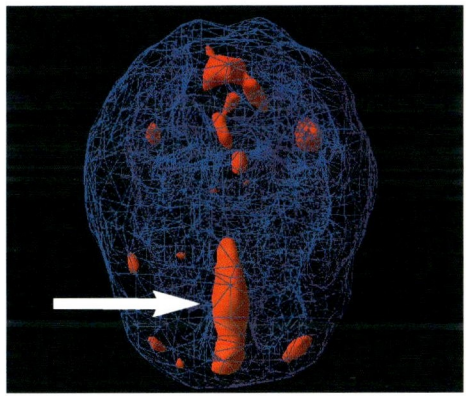
active top-down view

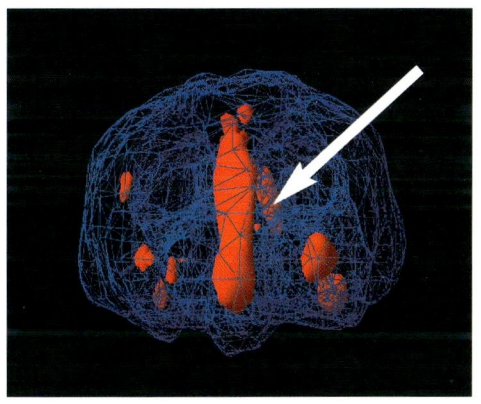
active front-on view

Functions

- allows shifting of attention
- cognitive flexibility
- adaptability
- helps the mind move from idea to idea
- gives the ability to see options
- helps you go with the flow
- cooperation

Problems

- worry
- holds onto hurts from the past
- stuck on thoughts (obsessions)
- stuck on behaviors (compulsions)
- oppositional behavior, argumentative
- uncooperative, tendency to say no
- addictive behaviors (alcohol or drug abuse, eating disorders, chronic pain)
- cognitive inflexibility
- obsessive compulsive disorder
- OCD spectrum disorders
- eating disorders, road rage

Functional Neuroanatomy

The Temporal Lobes

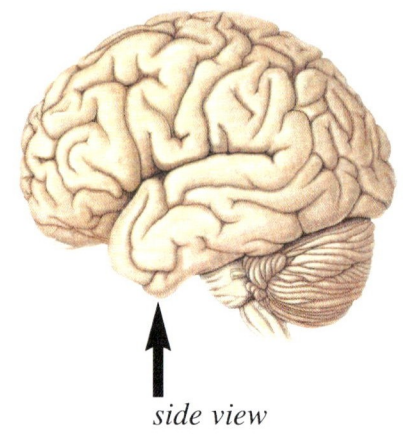
side view

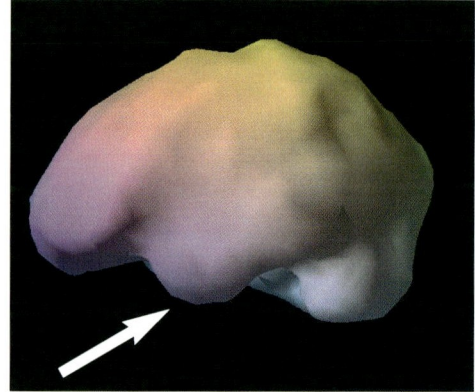
side surface view

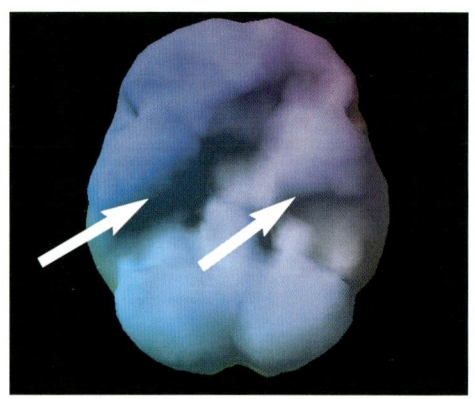
underside surface view

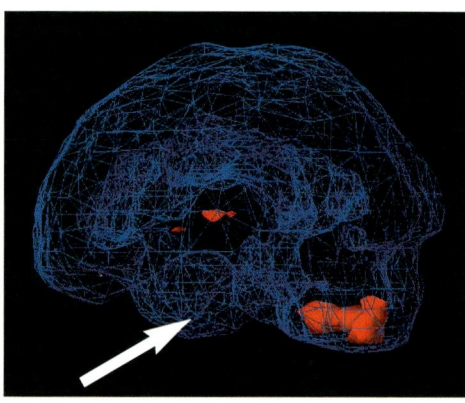
active side view

Functions

Dominant Side (usually the left)
- understanding and processing language
- intermediate-term memory
- long-term memory
- auditory learning
- retrieval of words
- complex memories
- visual and auditory processing
- emotional stability

Non-dominant Side (usually the right)
- recognizing facial expression
- decoding vocal intonation
- rhythm
- music
- visual learning

Problems

Dominant Temporal Lobe
- aggression, internally or externally driven
- dark or violent thoughts
- sensitivity to slights, mild paranoia
- word finding problems
- auditory processing problems
- reading difficulties
- emotional instability

Non-dominant Temporal Lobe
- difficuty recognizing facial expression
- difficulty decoding vocal intonation
- implicated in social skill struggles

Either/Both Temporal Lobe Problems
- memory problems, amnesia
- headaches or abdominal pain without a clear explanation
- anxiety or fear for no particular reason
- abnormal sensory perceptions, visual or auditory distortions
- feelings of déjà vu or jamais vu
- periods of spaciness or confusion
- religious or moral preoccupation
- hypergraphia, excessive writing
- seizures

Section 4

Images of Strokes
Compelling Reasons Not to Smoke!

Strokes are one of the leading causes of death in the U.S. They are caused by either a blood clot that chokes off blood supply to an area of the brain or by a blood vessel breaking. Cigarette smoking is one of the most significant risk factors for strokes. On SPECT, strokes are demonstrated by areas of significant decreased or absent activity. SPECT is often helpful in the evaluation and management of cerebral vascular disease. After an acute stroke, early SPECT depicts the area of ischemia with greater accuracy than either computed tomography or magnetic resonance imaging. When the perfusion defect is large, the likelihood of hemorrhagic complications or herniation increases. Reperfusion of an arterial territory after thrombolysis can be documented more conveniently with SPECT than with angiography. SPECT, before and after the injection of acetazolamide has been used to assess the vascular reserve in patients with severe stenosis of the proximal vessels of the cerebrovascular tree. Here are several examples.

Left Frontal Stroke

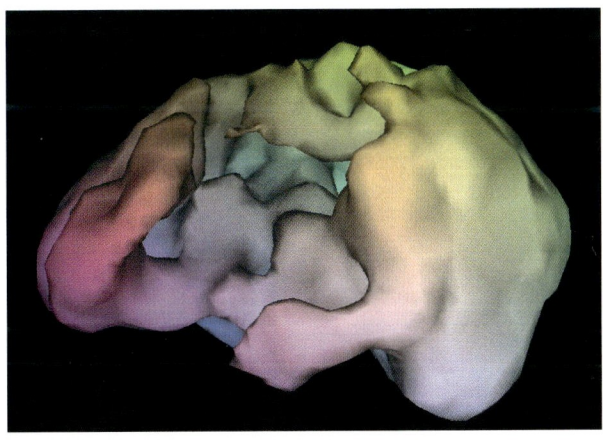

left side surface view

Ellen, 63, was suddenly paralyzed on the right side of her body. Unable to speak, she was in a panic and her family was extremely concerned. As drastic as these symptoms were, two hours after the event, her CAT scan was still normal. Suspecting a stroke, the emergency room physician ordered a brain SPECT study that showed a hole of activity in her left frontal lobe caused by a clot that had choked off the blood supply to this part of the brain. From this information, it was clear that a stroke had occurred and her doctors were able to take measures to limit the extent of the damage. Ellen was a smoker.

Left Frontal Stroke

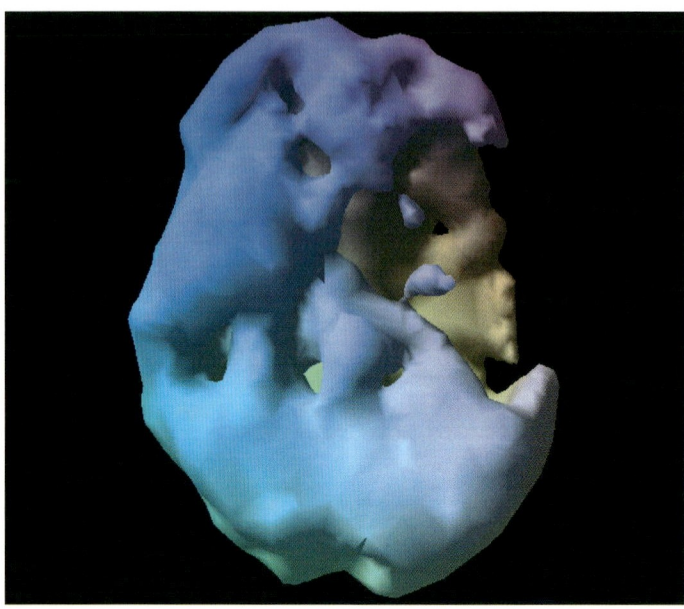

underside surface view

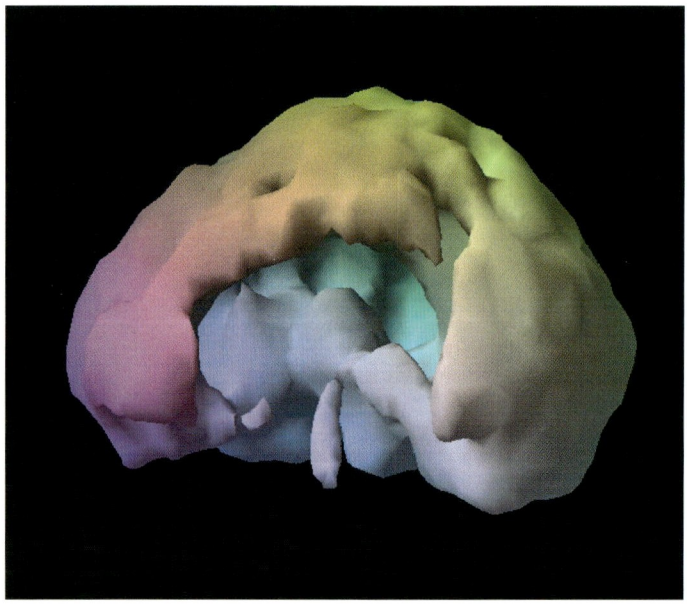

left side surface view

Bill, 48-year-old male with a left frontal lobe stroke, affecting speech, mood and temperament. Although Bill was not a cigarette smoker, he had over 10 years of moderate marijuana smoking.

Two Right Sided Strokes

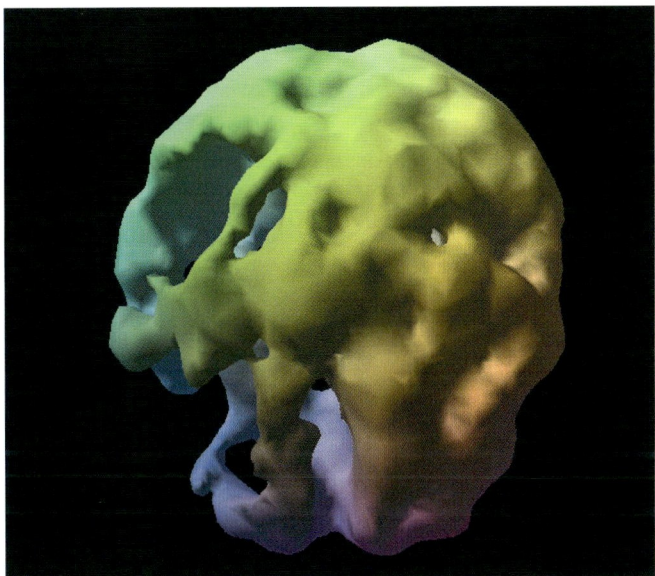

top down surface view

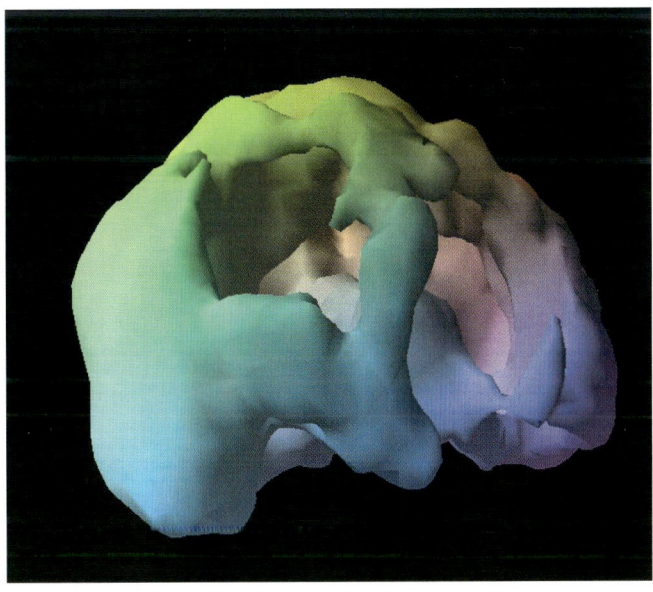

right side surface view

Nancy was a 59-year-old woman suffering from severe depression that had been unresponsive to treatment. Upon admission to a psychiatric hospital, a SPECT study was done to evaluate her condition. Since she had not experienced any symptoms that would indicate to this, I was surprised to see that she had had two large strokes. Almost immediately her unresponsive depression made more sense to me. Sixty percent of the people who have frontal lobe strokes experience severe depression within a year. As a result of the SPECT study, I sought immediate consultation with a neurologist who evaluated her for the possible causes of the stroke, such as plaque in the arteries of the neck or abnormal heart rhythms. He felt the stroke had come from blood clot and placed her on blood thinning medication to prevent further strokes. Nancy was a smoker.

Section 5

Images of Dementia vs Psuedodementia

As the population ages, the incidence of dementia in the U.S. will become an even more common problem and take up an even larger percentage of the health care budget. With the advent of new medications that slow the course of some dementing processes, diagnostic tools that help in the early differential diagnosis of dementia is essential. The SPECT pattern for Alzheimer's Disease is typically bilateral hypoperfusion in the parietal and temporal regions of the brain with frontal lobe hypoperfusion occurring later in the illness. Multi-infarct dementia is characterized by multiple areas of decreased perfusion. HIV dementia is typically seen by decreased patchy uptake across the cortex. Frontal lobe dementias (as the name indicates) are often characterized by very poor frontal lobe perfusion. Psuedodementia (another condition, such as depression, that clinically appears as dementia) will not have a typical dementia pattern and may be more like a depression pattern.

Here are several examples of how SPECT can be useful in the evaluation and treatment of dementia-like presentations

Alzheimer's Disease

bilateral decreased parietal and temporal lobe activity

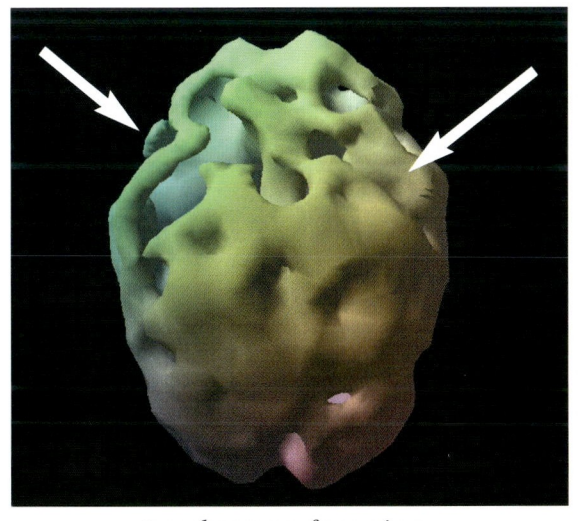 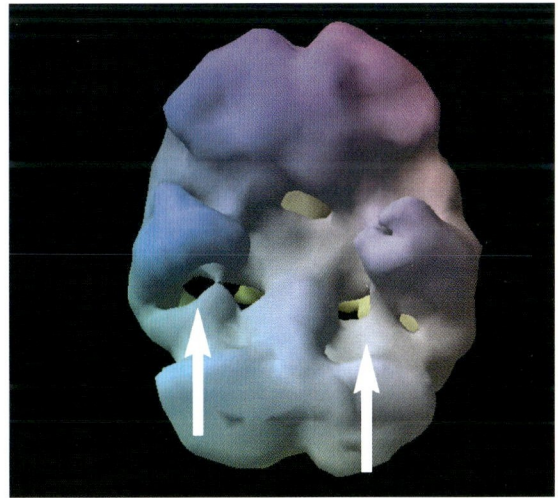

top-down surface view   *underside surface view*

When Frank, a wealthy, well-educated man, entered his seventies, he began to become forgetful. At first it was over small things, but as time went on the lapses of memory progressed to the point that he often forgot essential facts of his life: where he lived, his wife's name and even his own name. His wife and children, not understanding the change in behavior, were aggravated by his absent-mindedness and often angry at him for it. Frank's SPECT study showed a marked suppression across the entire brain, but especially in the frontal lobes, the parietal lobes and temporal lobes. This was a classic Alzheimer's disease pattern. By showing the family these images and pointing out the physiological cause of Frank's forgetfulness, in living images, I helped them understand that he was not trying to be annoying, but had a serious medical problem.

Consequently, instead of blaming him for his memory lapses, they began to show compassion towards him, and they developed strategies to deal, more effectively, with the problems of living with a person who has Alzheimer's Disease. In addition, I placed Frank on new experimental treatments for Alzheimer's Disease that seemed to slow the progression of the illness.

Alzheimer's Disease

Here is a scan of a 92-year-old man with Alzheimer's Disease who had become forgetful, frequently got lost away from home, forgot how to do simple things such as dress himself and began getting aggressive with his wife. Notice the extensive frontal lobe involvement.

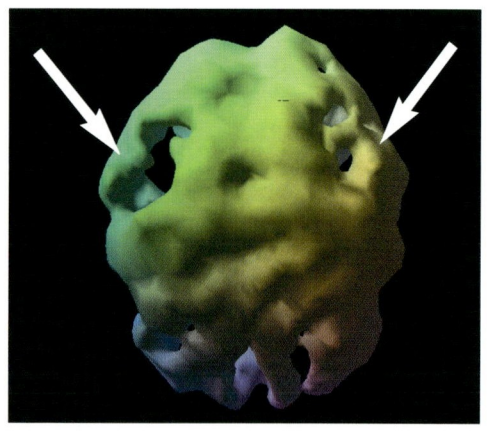
top-down surface view

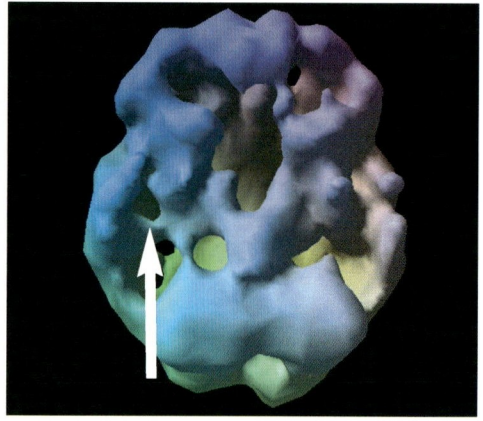
underside surface view

notice marked overall suppression, especially in the parietal lobes (arrows left images) and temporal lobes (arrows right image)

Pseudodementia

good temporal and parietal lobe perfusion, with increased limbic and/or decreased prefrontal cortex activity

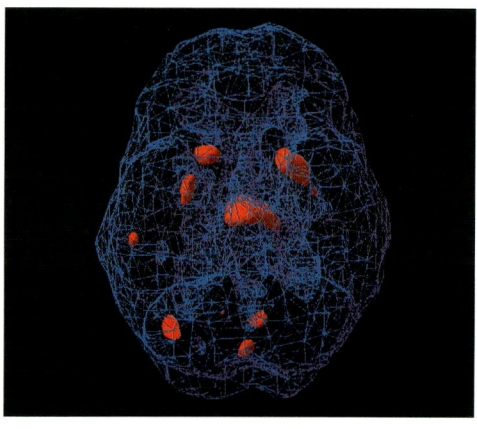
underside active view
before treatment

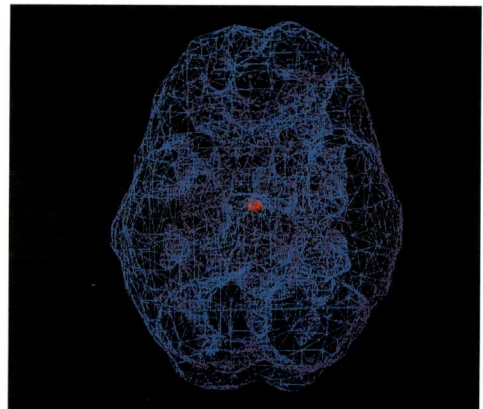
underside active view
after treatment

I first met Margaret when she was 68 years old. Her appearance was ragged and unkempt. She lived alone and her family was worried because she appeared to have symptoms of serious dementia. Her family finally admitted her to the psychiatric hospital at which I worked after she

Images of Dementia vs Psuedodementia

Section 6

Images of Brain Trauma

Wear a helmet, Avoid fights

No headers in soccer, Wear your seatbelt

Play golf instead of football

The impact of head trauma is often overlooked in psychiatry. Even minor head injuries to vulnerable parts of the brain can cause problems for years to come. SPECT is one of the best tools in evaluating functional deficits from head trauma that are often missed by other studies. This leads to more understanding and effective treatment for patients. Typically, SPECT findings in head trauma include focal areas of decreased activity, often in a contra-coup pattern (such as decreased activity in the left anterior prefrontal cortex and right occipital lobe or the anterior and posterior aspects of a temporal lobe) and, in some cases, marked hyperactivity over the site of the injury. In many cases we have seen increased "off center" cingulate gyrus activity after a head injury.

Documentation of head injuries is essential for several reasons. For school age children and teenagers it allows them to receive more specialized services. Knowledge of the injuries is often essential for legal/insurance reasons. Patient and family understanding of the effects of brain trauma enhances treatment compliance and a deeper understanding from family and support systems. Here are several examples.

Tim, age 15, was a high school sophomore at a high school in Connecticut. From a young age he exhibited severe conduct problems. He had already been arrested for shoplifting, he frequently cut school and was defiant and abusive toward his parents. He did not get along with other teens at school and seemed to "never fit in." He smoked a pack of cigarettes a day and frequently used both marijuana and cocaine. He had already been in one treatment program and was on his way to a second program when his parents brought him to our clinic. Since childhood, Tim was hyperactive, impulsive, moody and frequently angry, especially whenever someone would tell him no. His temper flared quickly and often, over minor or trivial incidences. He had tried numerous medications without success. His parents had heard about my clinic and decided to come across the country to see us.

His brain SPECT study showed severe damage to his left prefrontal cortex. It was one of the most severe cases I have ever seen. When he was 18 months old he fell down a flight of stairs. His mother said he was never quite the same since then. She could just tell there was a difference in his personality. Given the level of functional damage to Tim's brain I decided to put him on a combination of an anticonvulsant medication and a stimulant. It helped lessen the rage and improve his impulse control. Given the level of damage, his chances for full executive function are not very promising. The goal of treatment is to utilize every prescription available to help Tim develop auxiliary internal supervision mechanisms. Otherwise, legal authorities will have to impose external supervision in some form of a contained setting, basically through no fault of Tim. He doesn't have the capacity for internal supervision that is housed in the prefrontal cortex.

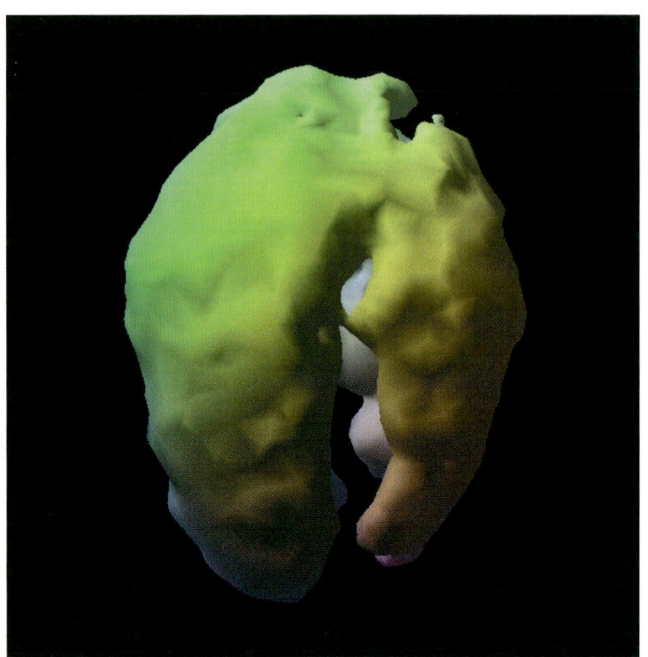
top down surface view

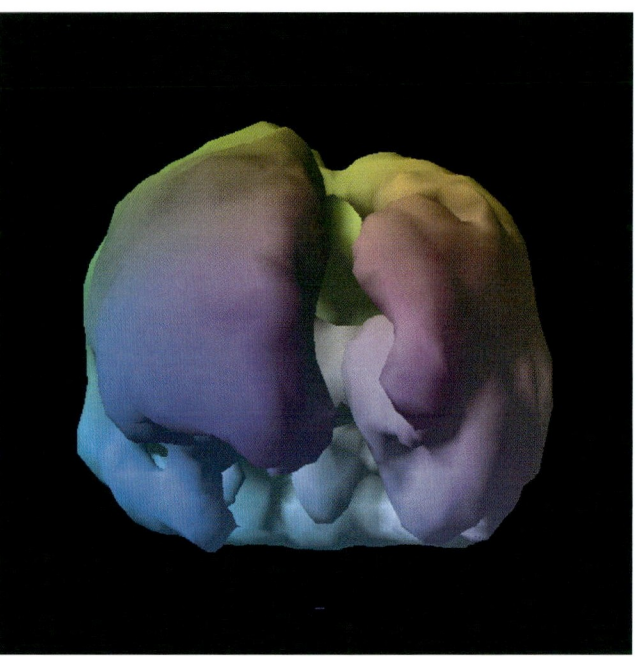
front on surface view

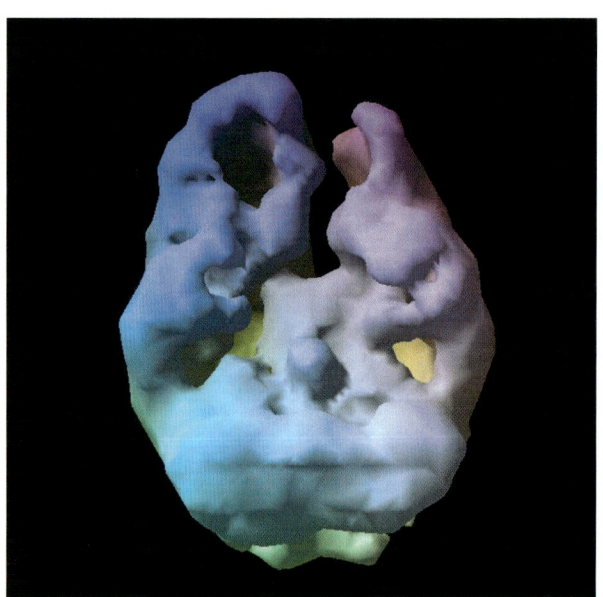
underside surface view

note the marked decreased left prefrontal, left hemisphere and left occipital lobe

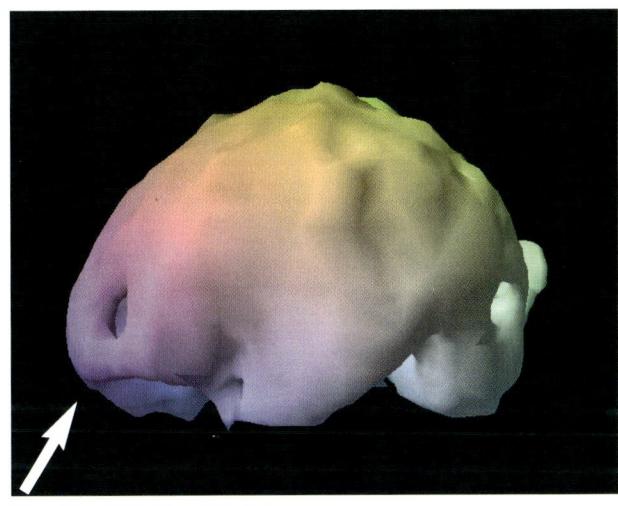

left side surface view

16 y/o-brain trauma at age 7, with school failure, substance abuse, impulsivity, decreased left pfc

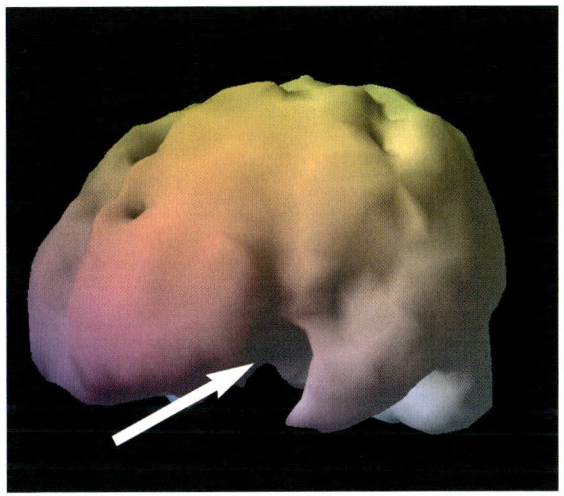

left side surface view

79 y/o-ran car into a pole at age 20, long history of aggression and irritability decreased left pfc and anterior temporal lobe

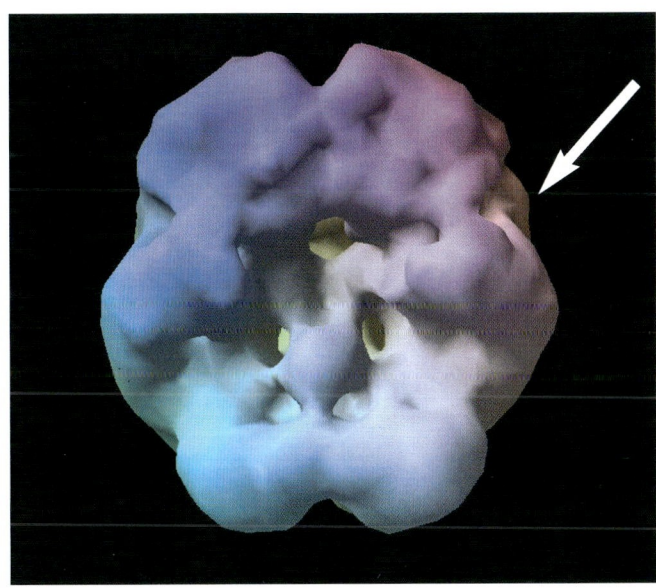

underside surface view

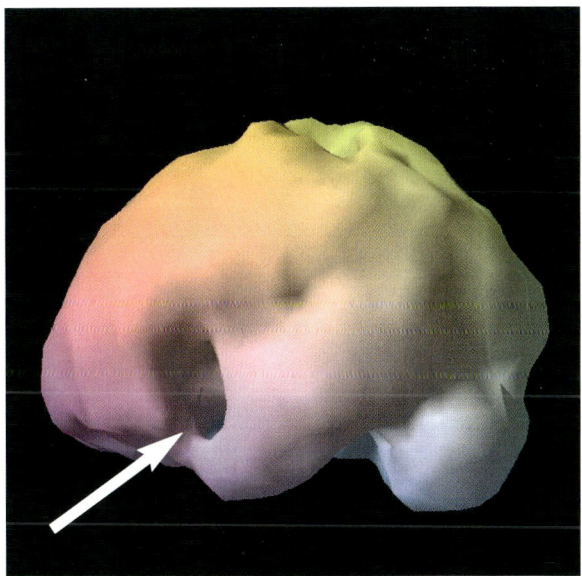

left side surface view

48 y/o male– football injury age 16, significant problems expressing feelings (alexythymia) decreased left pfc and anterior left temporal

Images of Brain Trauma

IMAGES OF HUMAN BEHAVIOR

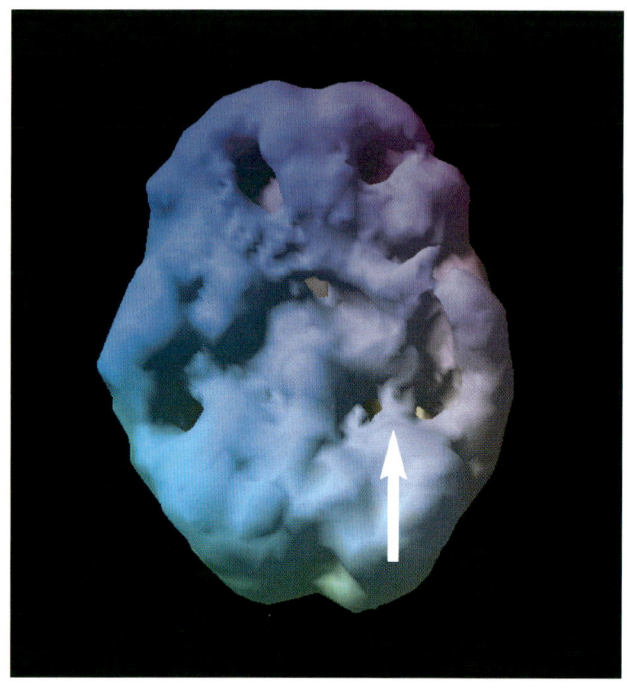

underside surface view 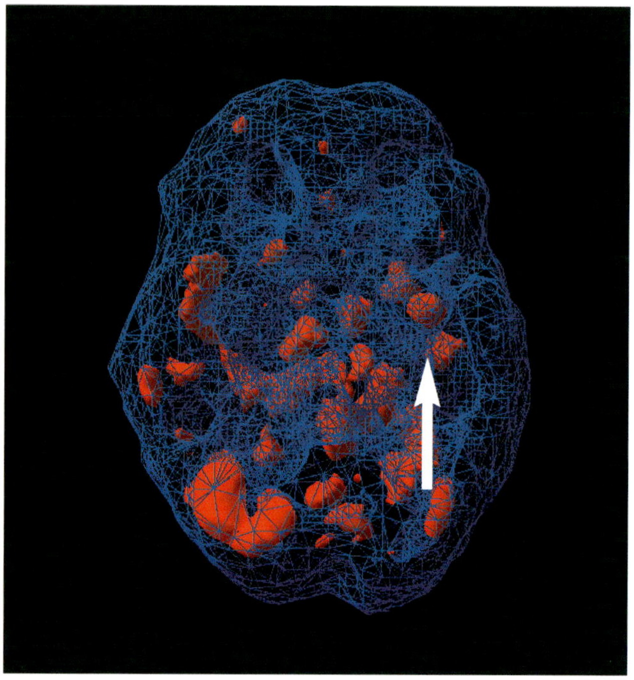   underside active view

56 y/o male–fell off porch into pile of bricks at age 6, significant problems with temper, illusions and depression; decreased left pfc and left temporal lobe (left image), increased deep left temporal lobe activity (right image)

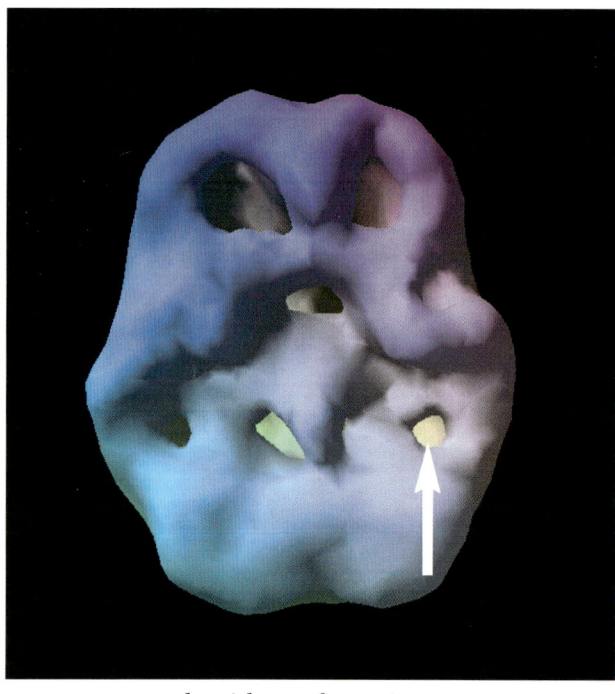 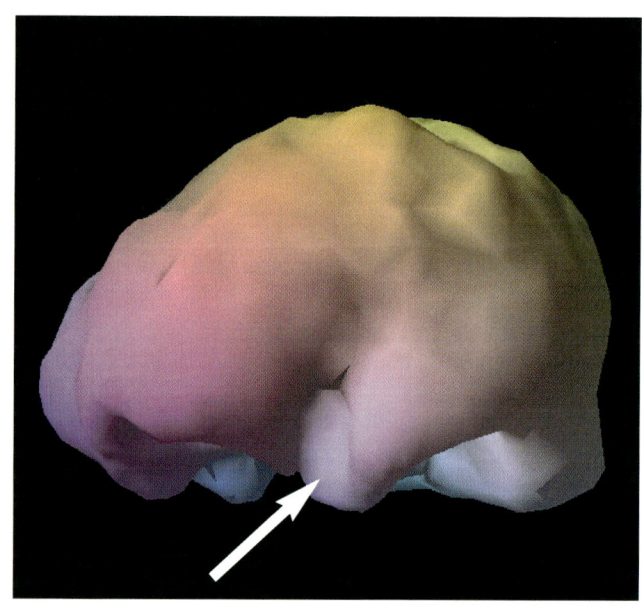

underside surface view   left side surface view

32 y/o female–rear ended by an 18 wheel semi-truck on the freeway, significant problems with irritability, depression and memory; decreased pfc and left temporal lobe (left image), decreased left anterior temporal lobe activity (right image)

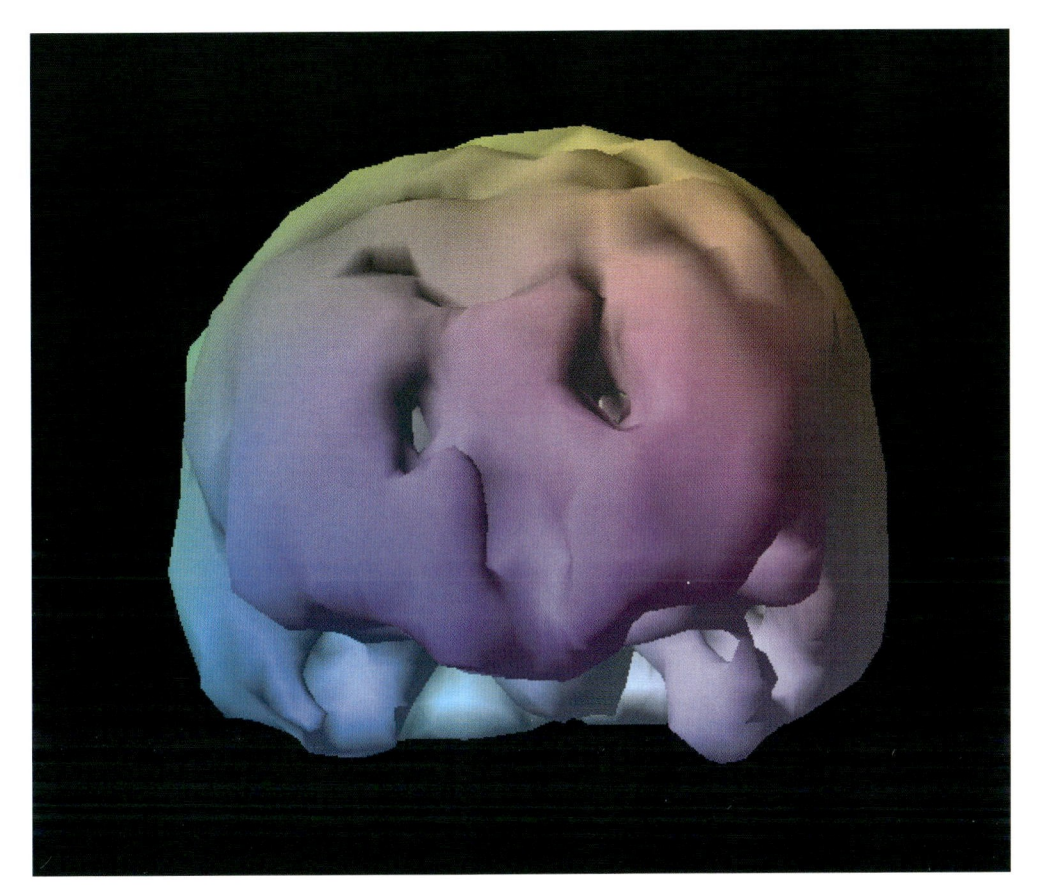

front on surface view
notice the dented area in the right anterior frontal pole

Betty was the most beautiful 88-year-old woman I had ever met. She was very proper and very proud. When she was a young woman she had emigrated from England after marrying a U.S. soldier. It was not her 90-year-old husband who brought her to the hospital to see me, however, it was her sister. Her husband, far from being supportive, angrily denied that his wife was suffering from serious cognitive problems. Yet during the evaluation process it was clear that Betty had severe memory problems; she did not know where she lived, her phone number, or her husband's name. I ordered a SPECT study that showed a dent in the right side of Betty's frontal lobe. It was obvious to me that she had, at some point in her life, suffered a significant head injury. When I asked her about it, all she could do was look down and cry; she could not give me details of the event. When I asked her sister, she reported that Betty and her husband had a stormy relationship and that he was abusive towards her. Sometimes he would grab her by the hair and slam her head into the wall. The sister wanted Betty to go to the police, but Betty said it would only make things worse.

Shortly after Betty was hospitalized, her husband began pressuring me to send her home. He kept protesting that there was nothing wrong with her, yet I knew that Betty needed to be removed from that environment so I contacted the Adult Protective Services. At Betty's hearing, I used her SPECT studies to convince the judge that her home held potential danger. He then ordered her to have a conservator, and she went to live with her sister.

Zachary, age 10, was a fun loving, active boy who was loving, sweet and liked to please. He did well in kindergarten and was liked by the other children. One summer, between kindergarten and first grade, Zachary was riding in the front seat of a car with his mother on a trip to his grandparents house. All of a sudden a drunk driver swerved into their lane causing the mother to quickly jerk the car to the side of the road. She lost control and the car hit a tree. The mother broke her leg in the accident and Zachary, in a seat belt, hit his head against the side window. Zachary was unconscious, but only for about 10 minutes.

Initially, they were glad to just be alive and Zachary and his mother became even closer than before. About six weeks later, however, Zachary's behavior began to change. He exhibited aggressive behavior, breaking his own toys and hurting his younger brother. He began swearing, which was a new behavior for him. He blurted out statements at inappropriate times and interrupted frequently. He became rude, contrary, argumentative and conflict seeking. He lost his friends at school the next year because he would say things that would hurt their feelings. He started to tease the two cats at home, so much so that they started to avoid him whenever he came into the house. Six months after the accident his mother knew that there was something seriously the matter. She brought him to a counselor who thought the problem was psychological, as a result of the accident. The counselor thought that Zachary and his mother were too close and developed strategies to help Zachary become more independent. That only seemed to make things worse. After two years of counseling, which didn't seem to help much, the mother consulted Zachary's her pediatrician. He diagnosed Zachary with ADD and put him on Ritalin. But it didn't help very much. In fact, it only seemed to make him more aggressive. When Zachary was brought to me at age 9, I thought he might have a chronic post concussive syndrome, secondary to the accident. His brain SPECT study revealed marked decreased activity in the left pfc and decreased activity in the left occipital cortex, indicating both a front and back injury (common in head injuries). In addition, he had decreased activity in his left temporal lobe. Given this constellation of findings I put him on a combination of medication (an anticonvulsant, to stabilize his aggressiveness and help his temporal lobe function, and amantadine [Symmetrel] to help with focus, concentration and impulse control). He was also placed in a special class at school and given cognitive retraining exercises. Over the next several months his behavior began to improve and he was able to live at home.

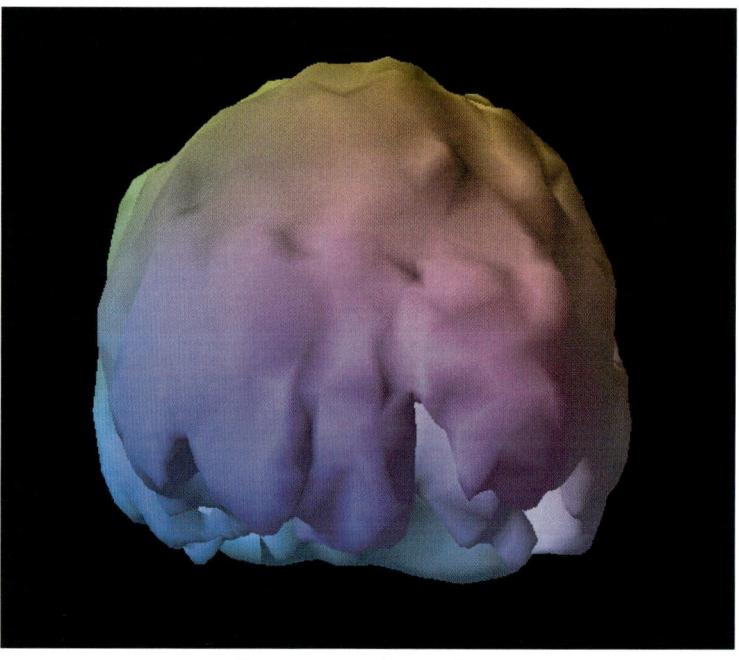

front on surface view
notice the dented area in the left anterior frontal pole

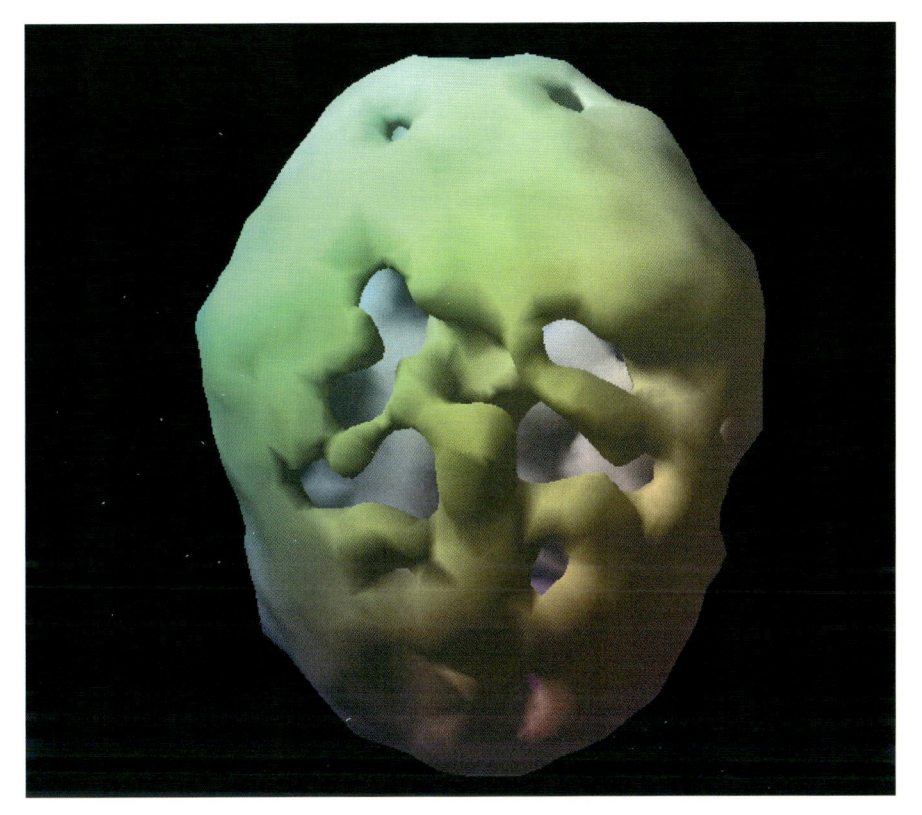

top down surface view
notice marked overall decreased activity
43 y/o male–motorcycle accident

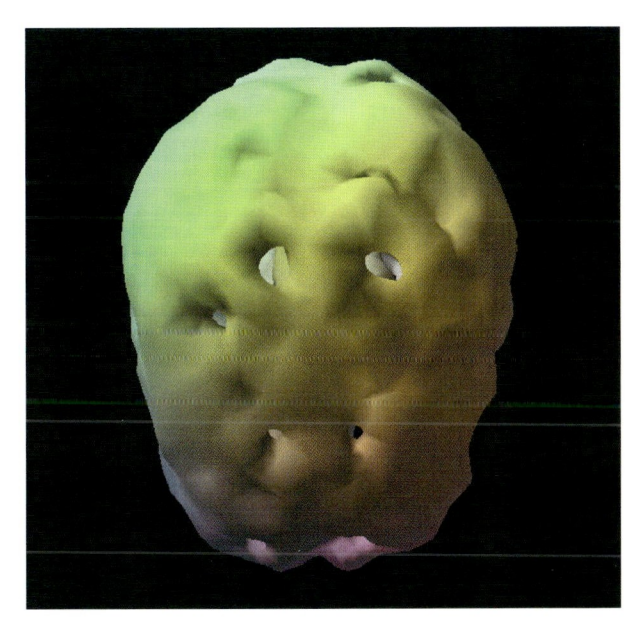

28 y/o male–bicycle accident, no helmet
problems with impulsivity and concentration

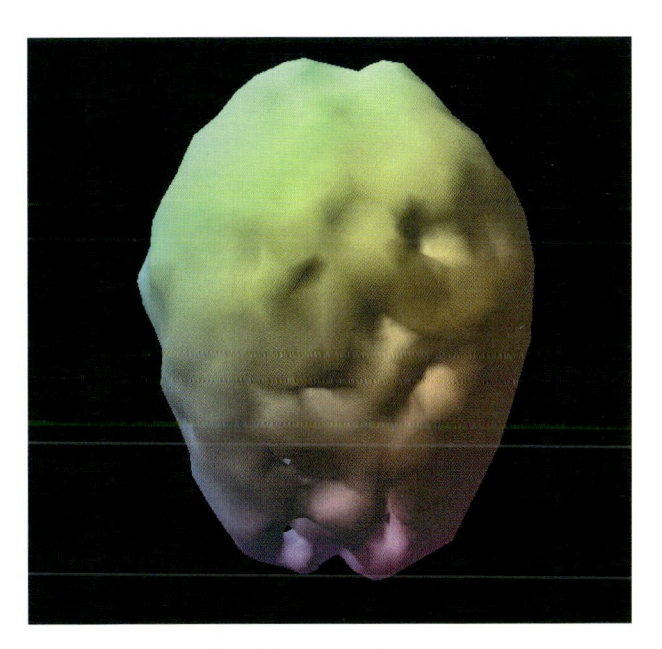

26 y/o–rollerblade accident, no helmet
executive function problems, suicidal ideas

Images of Brain Trauma

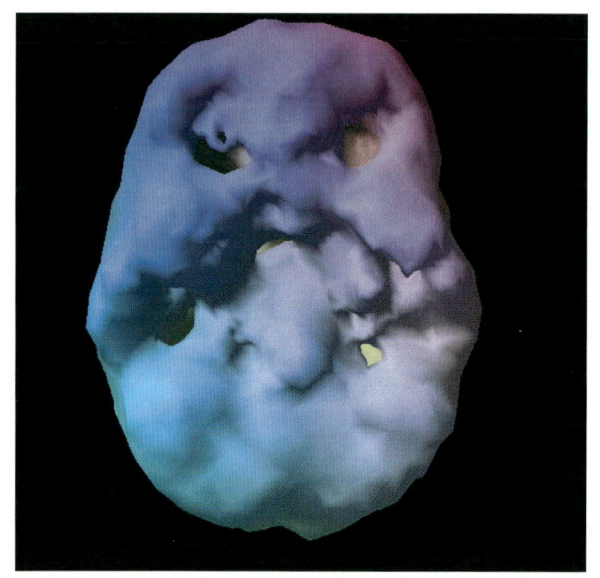

underside surface view

15 y/o–horseback riding accident
memory, concentration and school problems

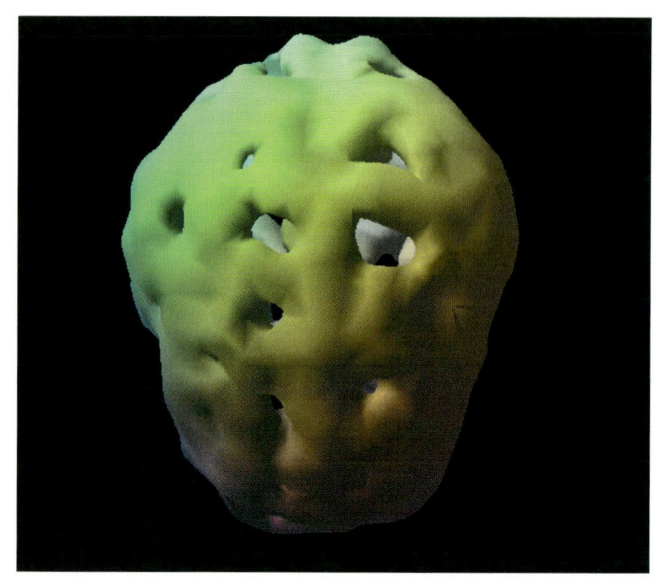

top down surface view

26 y/o–bar fight, hit with large mirror
executive function problems, note contra coup
injury to frontal and occipital lobes

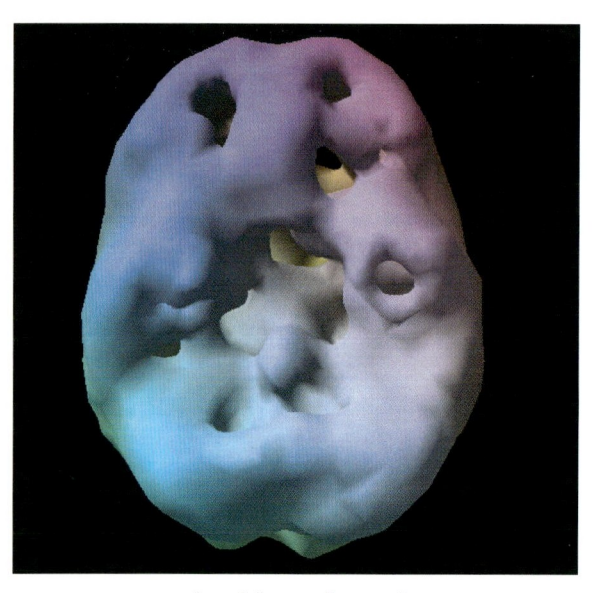

underside surface view

62 y/o–fall from a ladder

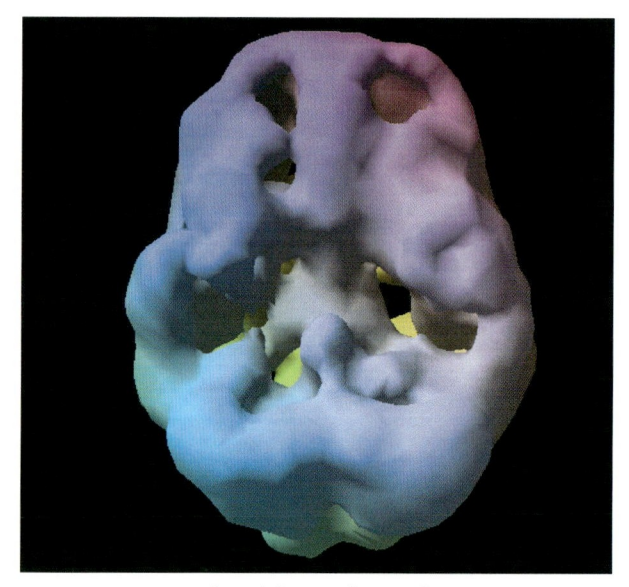

underside surface view

36 y/o–car accident

Images of Brain Trauma

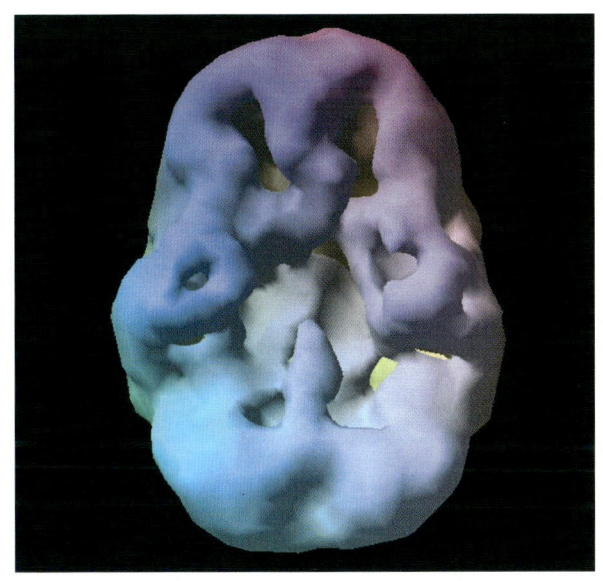

severe memory problems
underside surface view

22 y/o–diving accident
memory, concentration and mood problems

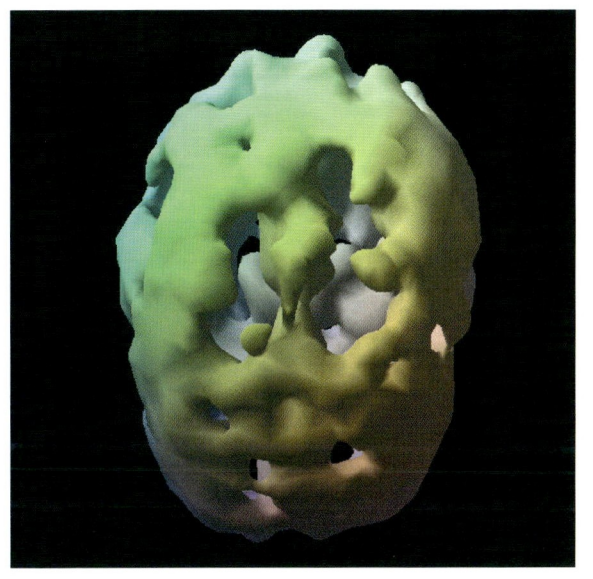

memory and temper problems
top down surface view

16 y/o–fell down stairs at age 3
school failure, aggression, in jail for rape

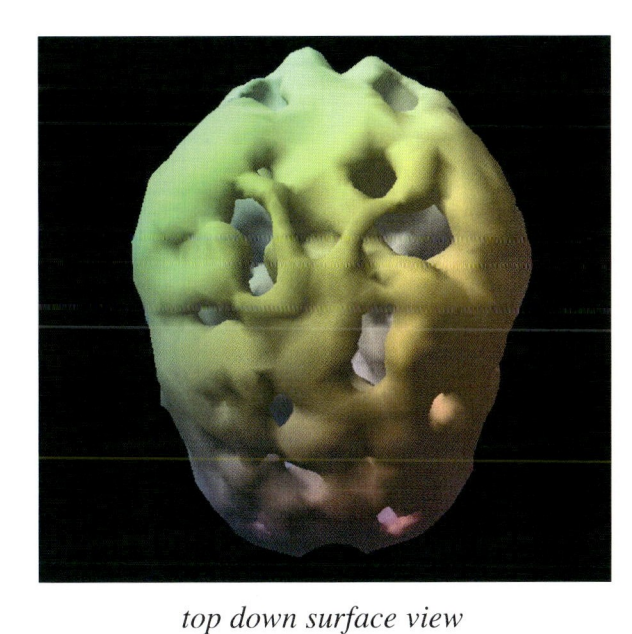

top down surface view

21 y/o–tackle football concussion
aggression problems

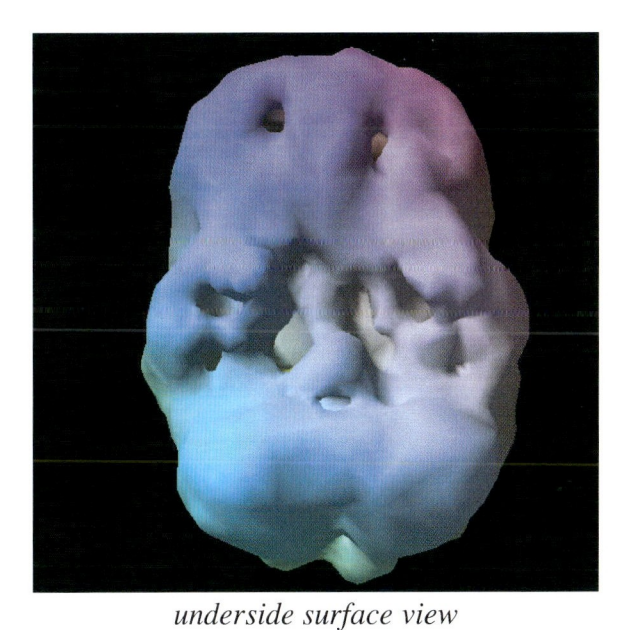

underside surface view

10 y/o–fell off jungle gym
school failure, temper problems

Images of Brain Trauma

Fall from Roof

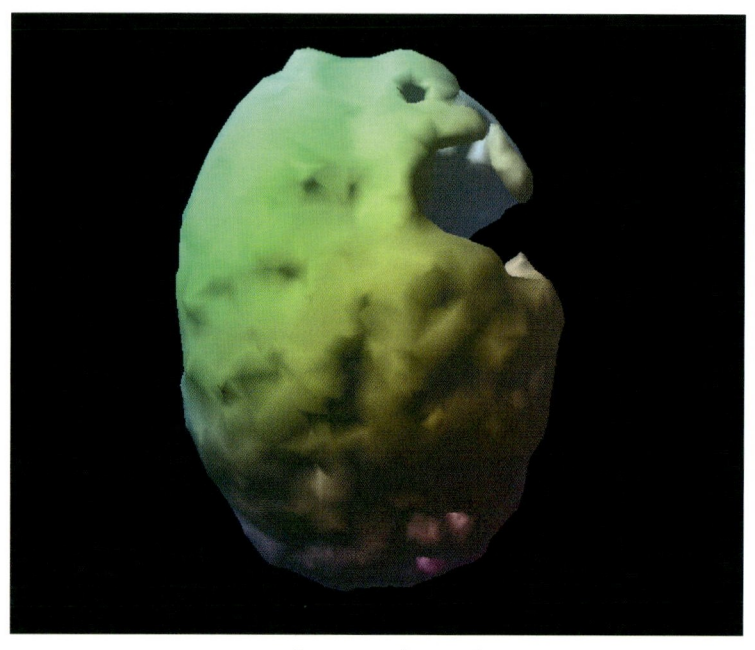

top down surface view
note large defect left parietal area

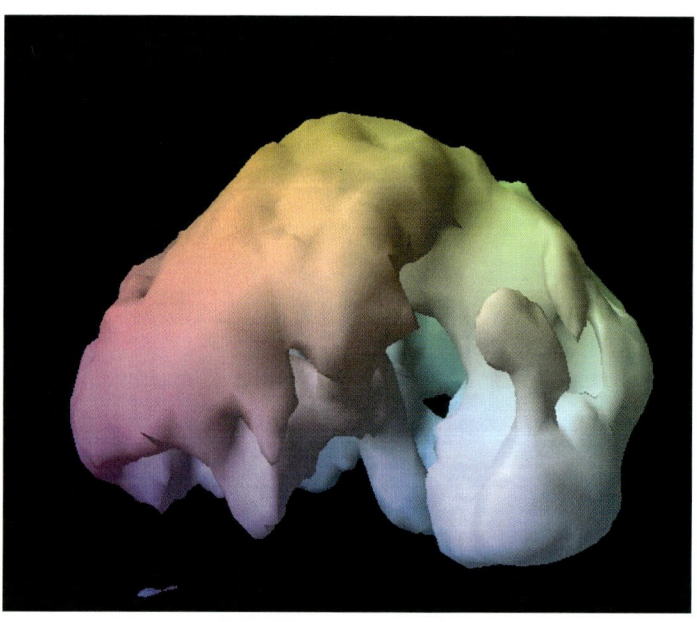

left side surface view
note large defect left parietal and temporal lobe area

48-year-old male roofer who fell 25 feet off a roof. Subsequently, he had problems with speech, attention, memory, concentration and temper. His wife divorced him.

24 Year Old Female Fall From Third Story

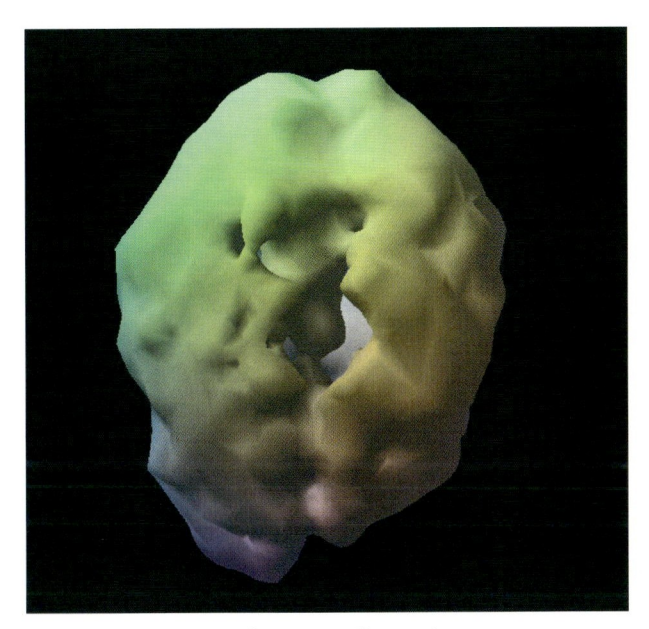

top down surface view
note marked decreased prefrontal activity

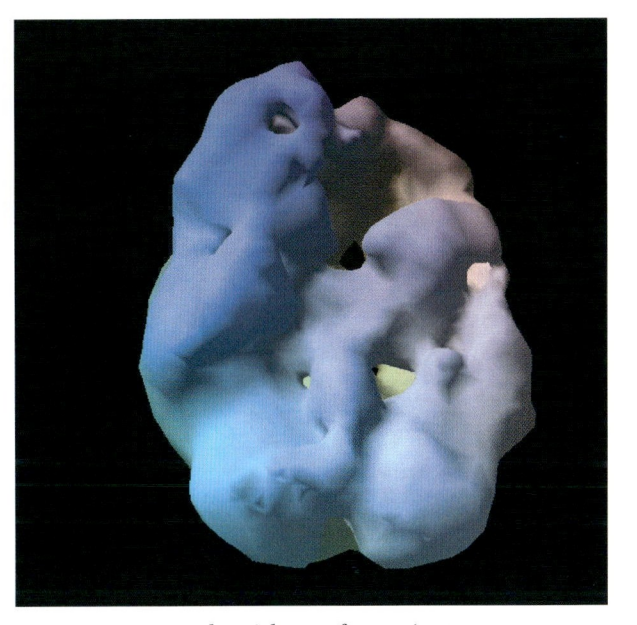

underside surface view
marked overall decreased activity

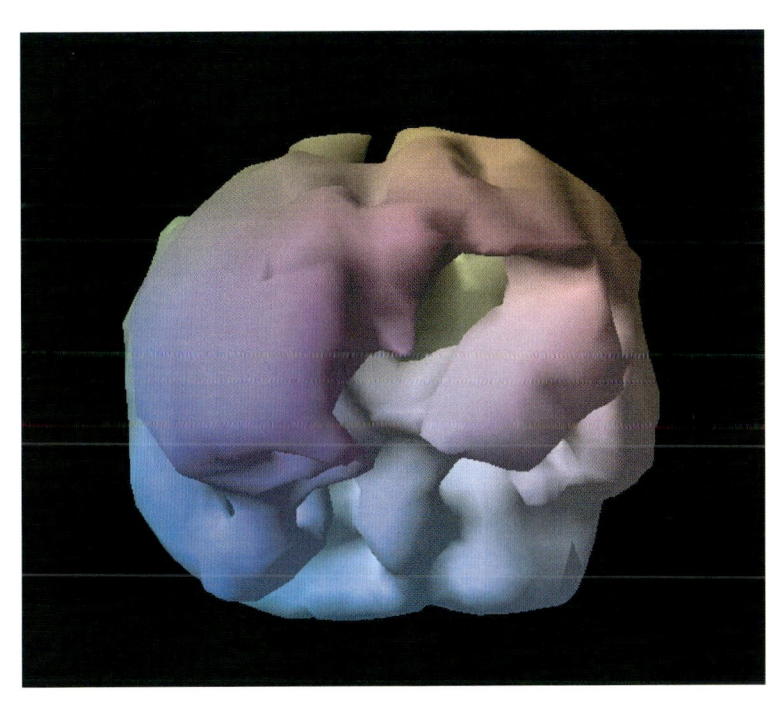

front on view
marked decreased prefrontal area

Images of Depression

Decreased prefrontal cortex activity at rest, especially on the left side, is a consistent SPECT finding in depression. The severity of depression is often related to the degree of frontal hypometabolism. Several studies have indicated that the hypometabolism normalizes after treatment if the patient's mood improved. Research indicates increased limbic system activity correllates with depression (thalamus, amygdala, cingulate gyrus and deep temporal lobes). When depressed patients perform a concentration task the left prefrontal cortex often activates to normal levels, differentiating depression from attention deficit disorder, which often shows normal activity at rest and decreased prefrontal cortex activity with concentration.

SPECT can be helpful in the diagnosis and treatment of complex or resistant depressive disorders by differentiating them from other disorders. This enhances patient compliance as the patient is able to "see the changes in the brain," and by subtyping depression. Here are three subtypes that I have identified.

- Decreased prefrontal cortex activity with increased deep limbic system (thalamus) activity. This subtype is often associated with moodiness, negativity, low energy, sleep, appetite problems and poor concentration. It often responds best to dopaminergic or noradrenergic interventions such as buprion, imipramine or desipramine.

- Increased anterior cingulate (this part of the brain is heavily innervated with serotonergic nerve fibers), thalamus and basal ganglia activity. This subtype is often associated with sadness, negativity, irritability, worry, cognitive inflexibility and getting stuck or locked into negative thought patterns. It often responds best to the serotonergic antidepressants such as fluoxetine, sertraline, paroxetine and venlafaxine.

- Decreased prefrontal cortex activity with increased or decreased temporal lobe activity. This is often the most serious subtype and it is often associated with sadness, irritability, rage (toward others or self in suicidal behavior), mild paranoia, atypical pain (atypical headaches or abdominal pain) and insomnia. I have seen this subtype made significantly worse by serotonergic medications and it is often helped by anticonvulsants, such as gabapentin or divalproate.

1. Decreased prefrontal cortex activity with increased deep limbic system activity.

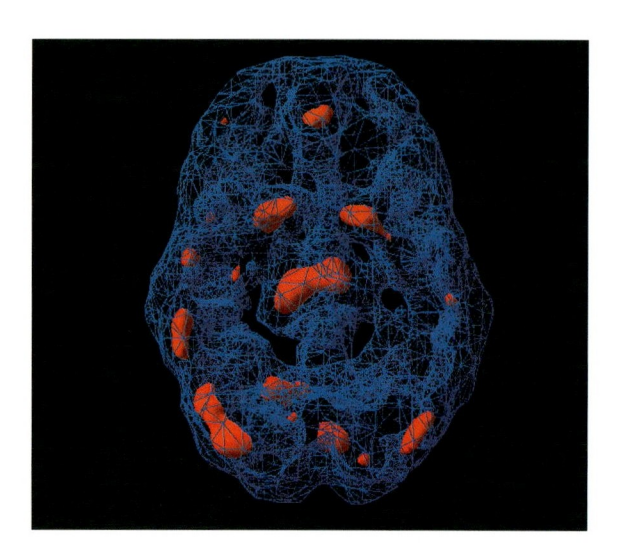

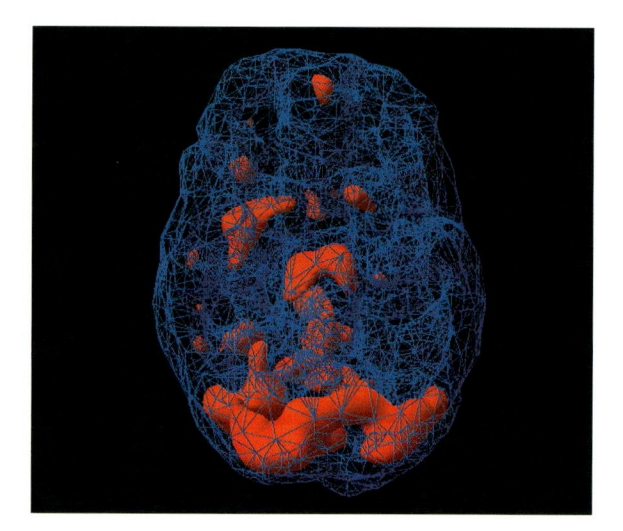

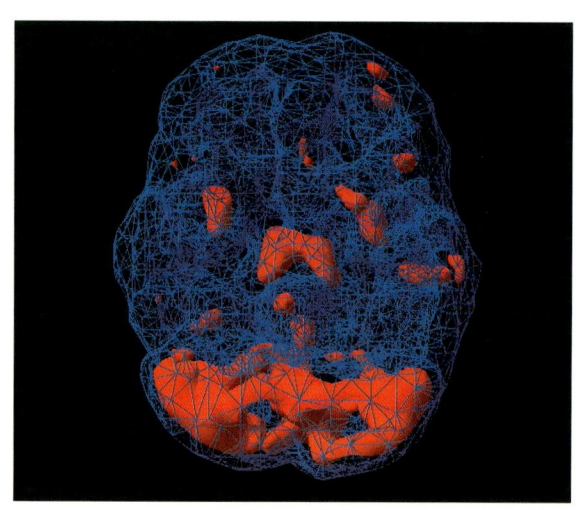

underside active views
notice increased deep limbic activity

Here is an example of deep limbic dysfunction. Leigh Anne came to see me fifteen months after the birth of her first child. Several weeks after her child was born she began experiencing symptoms of nausea, social withdrawal, crying spells and depression. Three months later she sought help through psychotherapy. But her condition did not improve. Her depression progressed to the point where she became unable to care for her daughter on a day-to-day basis. Desperate to function as the good mother she wanted to be to her child, she came to see me. After diagnosing her with major depression I placed her on Prozac and began seeing her in psychotherapy. Her symptoms remitted after only several weeks. After several months Leigh Anne discontinued treatment. She associated taking Prozac with a course of action for "a depressed person." She did not want to see herself in that light or be stigmatized with that label. For several months after stopping she had no adverse reaction, however, the symptoms eventually returned.

When she came to see me again Leigh Anne still didn't want to believe that anything was "wrong" with her, so she was still resistant to going back on medication. After I ordered a brain study to evaluate her deep limbic system, I was able to point out the marked increase in activity in that area of her brain. It provided me with the evidence needed to convince her to go back on Prozac for a while longer.

This case illustrates an important point. It has been my experience, as well as that of many other psychiatrists, that a patient does not necessarily have to stay on medication forever just because they have started it. However, with certain medications, like Prozac, a minimum period of treatment is necessary before it can successfully be terminated. If a depressed patient is willing to stay on their medication for long enough, about two years in this case, there is a greater chance that they can get off of it in a timely manner and remain symptom free.

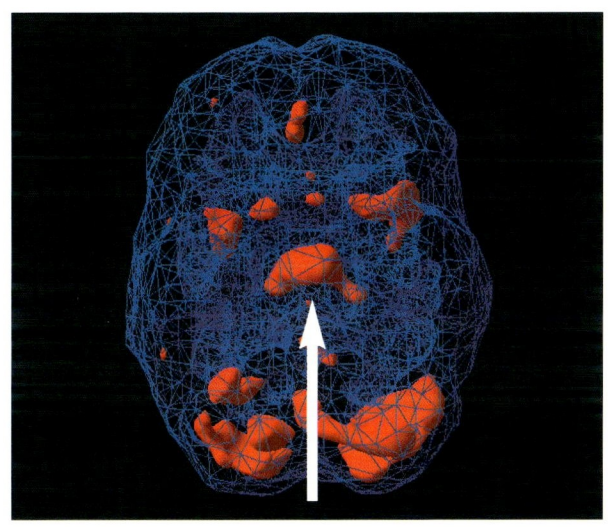

underside active view
notice increase limbic activity (arrow)

2. Increased anterior cingulate (this part of the brain is heavily innervated with serotonergic nerve fibers), thalamus and basal ganglia activity.

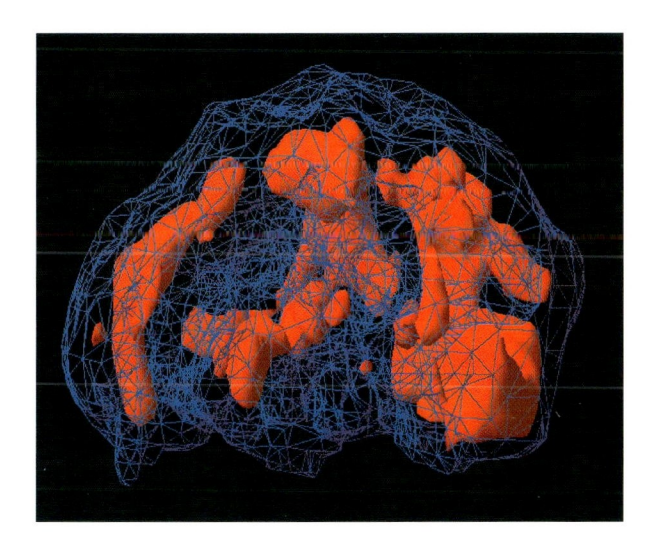

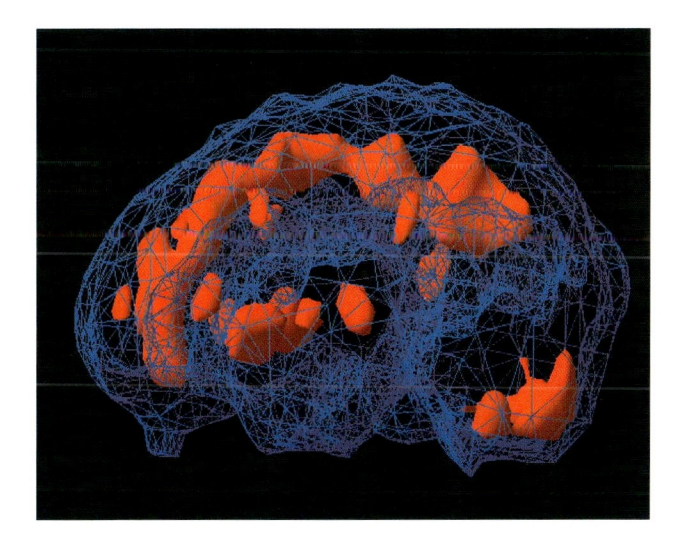

left side active views
notice increased cingulate, deep limbic and basal ganglia activity

3. Decreased prefrontal cortex activity with increased or decreased temporal lobe activity.

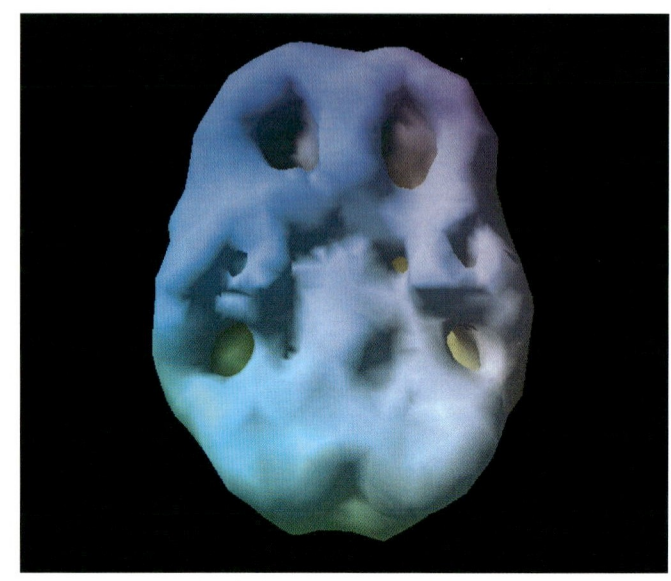

underside surface view marked decreased prefrontal and temporal lobe activity

Cindy is a 17-year-old who presented with symptoms of depression, suicidal thoughts and severe irritability. Serotonergic medications increased her irritability, depression and suicidal thoughts. Her SPECT study showed marked decreased activity in the left temporal lobe and prefrontal cortex. She responded positively to a combination of Lamictal and Wellbutrin and psychotherapy.

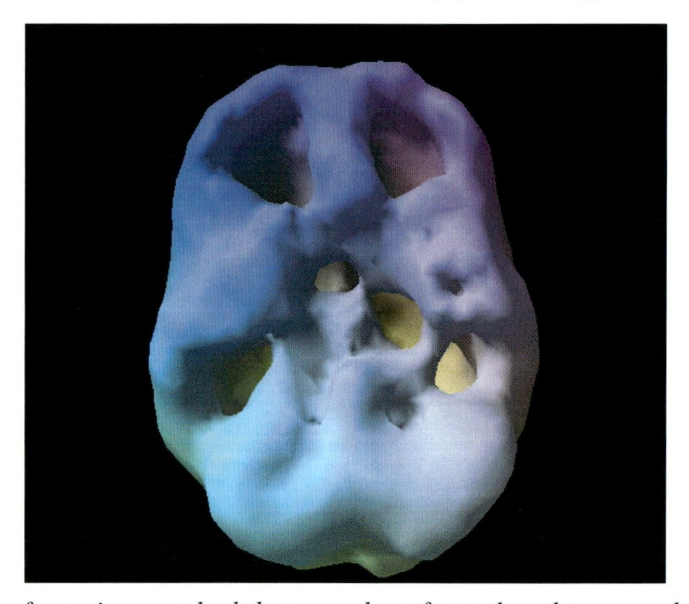

underside surface view marked decreased prefrontal and temporal lobe activity

Summer is an 18-year-old female who came for evaluation after an overdose of pills combined with alcohol in a suicide attempt. She had 4 prior suicide attempts along with a history of drug abuse, run away behavior, aggressive outbursts and school failure. Her SPECT study showed marked decreased activity in the left temporal lobe and prefrontal cortex bilaterally. She responded positively to a combination of Tegretol and desipramine and psychotherapy.

SECTION 8

Images of Bipolar Disorder and Schizophrenia

Bipolar disorder has been characterized by increased activity across the cerebral cortex. Clinically, during the manic phase, the scans often look hyperactive, especially in the lateral frontal cortex, lateral parietal lobes and lateral temporal lobes; focal increased uptake in the limbic system has also been noted. Differentiating the initial onset of bipolar disorder from schizophrenia is often a difficult task in an acutely psychotic individual. In schizophrenia SPECT findings have frequently reported decreased activity, especially in the prefrontal cortex. SPECT studies may provide helpful information in the differential diagnoses of these disorders. In addition, SPECT can provide useful information to patients to significantly improve compliance in disorders where compliance is a frequent serious problem. Here are several examples.

Bipolar Disorder

Sarah was fifty-three years old when she was admitted to the hospital under my care. The month before, her family had her committed to another psychiatric hospital for delusional thinking and bizarre behavior – she had actually ripped out all the electrical wiring in her home because she heard voices coming from the walls. In addition to the above symptoms, she was barely getting any sleep, her thoughts raced wildly, and she was irritable. In the previous hospital her doctor had diagnosed her with manic-depressive disorder (a cyclical mood disorder). He had placed her on lithium (an anti-manic medication) and an anti-anxiety medication. After responding well, she was sent home. But Sarah, like Leigh Anne, did not want to believe that anything was wrong with her and she stopped taking both medications. Her position was actually fortified by some members of her family who openly told her she didn't need pills, that doctors only prescribe them to force patients into numerous follow-up visits. Yet their advice was ill advised, for within weeks of stopping the treatment, Sarah's bizarre behavior returned. This was when her family brought her to the hospital where I worked. When I first saw Sarah, she was extremely paranoid. Believing that everyone was trying to hurt her, she was always looking for ways to escape the hospital. Again her thoughts were delusional; she believed she had special powers and that others were trying to take them from her. At times, she also appeared very "spacey." In an attempt to understand what was going on with her for myself, and to convince her that her problems were biological, I ordered a SPECT study.

Carrying out the scan did not prove easy. Our clinic tried to scan her on three separate occasions. The first two times she ripped out the intravenous line saying we were trying to poison her. The third time was a success because her sister went with her and calmed her down by talking her through the experience. While the study revealed an overall increase in activity in the deep limbic system, I found more intensity on the left side of her scan (focal increased deep limbic uptake) and a marked patchy uptake across the cortex. In other words, some areas showed increased activity and some showed decreased. My experience told me that cyclic mood disorders often correlate, specifically, with focal areas of increased activity in the deep limbic system as well as a patchy uptake across the surface of the brain in general.

For Sarah's family, this was powerful evidence that her problems were biological, so that when she still refused medication, they were now willing to encourage her to go back on it. After she took their advice, her behavior normalized again and once I knew she was feeling better, more in control, I showed her the brain studies. Through a better understanding of the problem she was able to agree to follow-up visits and to stay on her medication until both she and I concurred that she could stop.

Sometimes I'll rescan a patient several months after the initial scan to see what difference the medication has made on the physiology of his or her brain. Although Sarah's new study showed a vast improvement from her earlier one, I still noticed an area of increased activity in the left temporal lobe, and Sarah was still complaining of symptoms of spaciness. I changed her medication to Depakote, which is primarily used as an anti-seizure medication, but has also been used for manic-depressive disorder. Not only did her psychotic symptoms remain in remission but the spaciness disappeared as well. Five years later only a small dose of Depakote has given Sarah a normal life

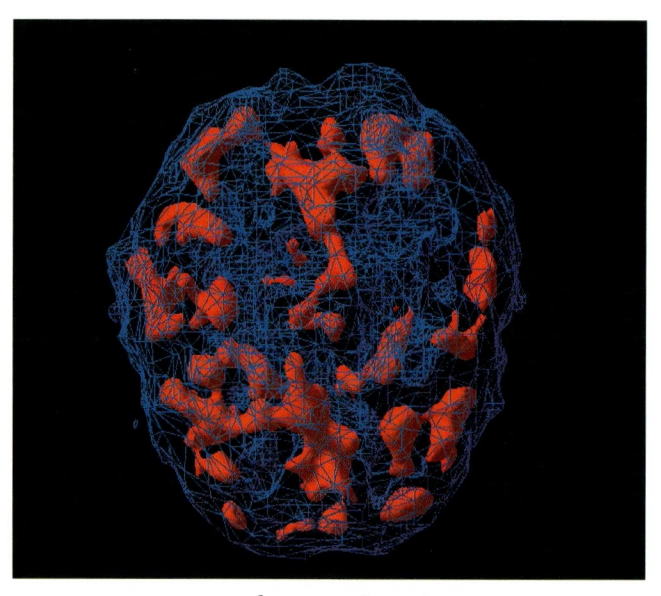

top-down active view
note patchy uptake throughout the cortex

Sarah's case illustrates one of the most clinically significant problems in people diagnosed with manic-depressive illness. This disorder is usually quite responsive to medication. The problem is that when people afflicted by the disorder improve, they feel so normal they do not believe they ever had a chronic problem to begin with. It is difficult for people to accept that they have to keep taking medication when they think they no longer have a problem. Yet, as we have seen, prematurely stopping medication actually increases their chances for relapse. Through the use of these brain studies I have been able to decrease the relapse rate of my patients by demonstrating, graphically, the biological nature of their disorders and the need to treat them as such. It has been a great asset to me in getting patients to cooperate in their own healing process. In addition, it has helped me with one other important thing: convince patient's to stop blaming themselves for their symptoms. Here are two more sets of images of bipolar patients taken during the manic phase of the illness.

Ryan was a 20-year-old male who presented with symptoms of grandiosity, racing thoughts, decreased sleep, irritability and agitation. His parents reported there was a family history of bipolar disorder in his grandfather.

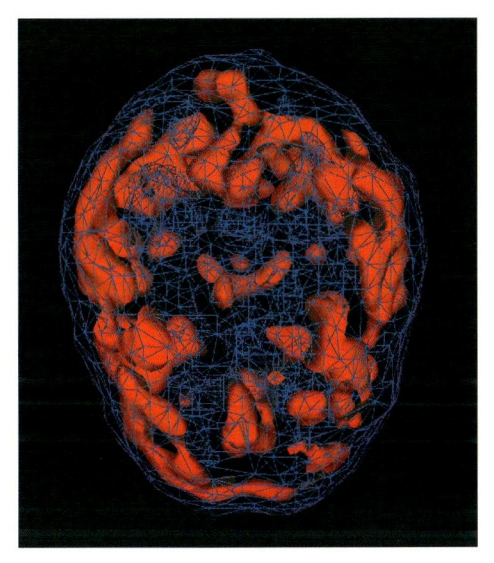

top down active view

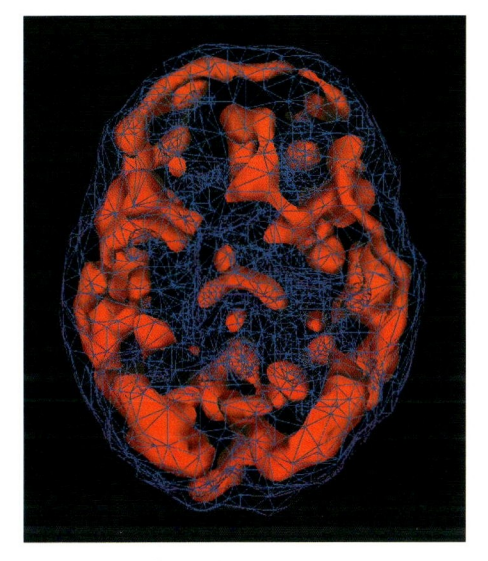

underside active view

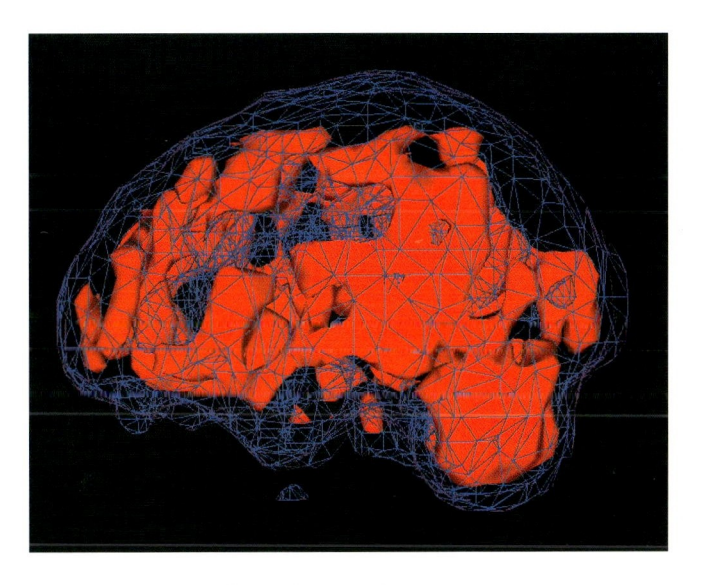

left side active view
note the marked increased patchy uptake throughout the cerebral cortex

Carrie was a second year college student when she first began having problems. She would go days without sleeping. She began having trouble concentrating in school and stopped going to classes. She started having sexual relationships with 4 different men and she spent all of the money she had for the school year in three months. When her parents discovered the problems they brought her in for evaluation. Carrie did not feel that anything was wrong. She felt that she had just made several poor decisions, like anyone her age. Her parents felt things were not the same. She had always been a thoughtful, responsible person prior to the last several months. A scan was ordered to help evaluate the clinical situation. It revealed marked patchy uptake throughout the cortex. Lithium was very helpful for Carrie and she was able to return to school the next semester.

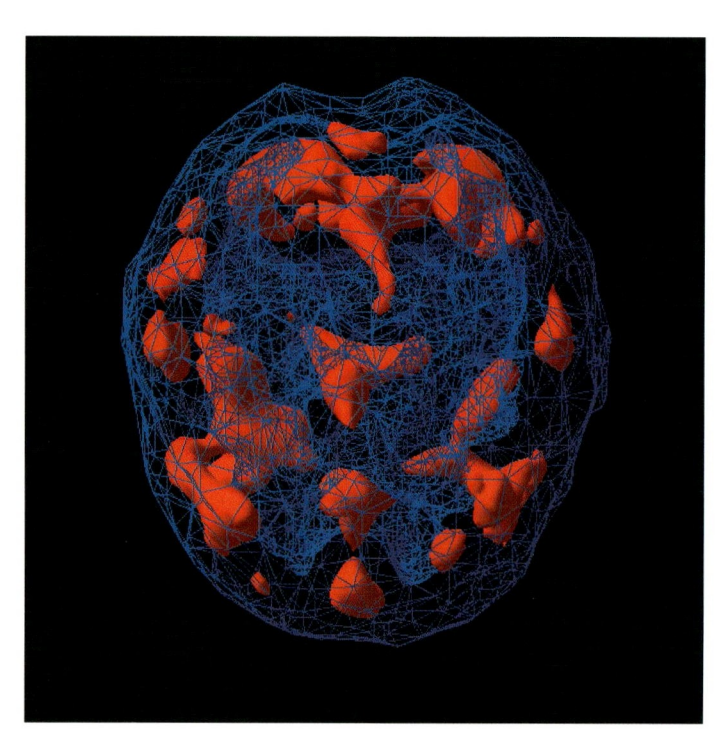

3D top-down active view
patchy increased uptake across the cortical surface

Schizophrenia

A 35-year-old man who had been living on the street was brought for evaluation by his mother. He had previously been diagnosed on many occassions with paranoid schizophrenia, but refused medication. His SPECT study revealed marked overall decreased activity throughout the cerebral cortex. Being able to see his own brain activity, represented by the 3D surface SPECT study, was helpful for him. He agreed to take his medication under his mother's supervision. One month later, after significant clinical improvement on 4 mg of risperidone a repeat SPECT study was performed. It showed improved overall cerebral perfusion. Being able to see the before and after SPECT studies side by side on the imaging computer monitor again was very encouraging to the patient and helped significantly with compliance.

Paranoid Schizophrenia, before and after treatment with risperidone

(top-down and underside surface views)

Before Treatment

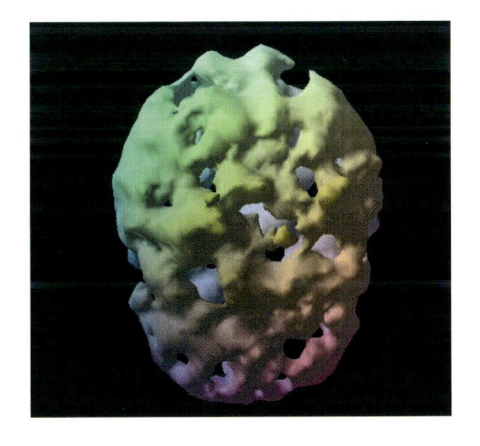

After Treatment

marked decreased activity throughout the cerebral cortex

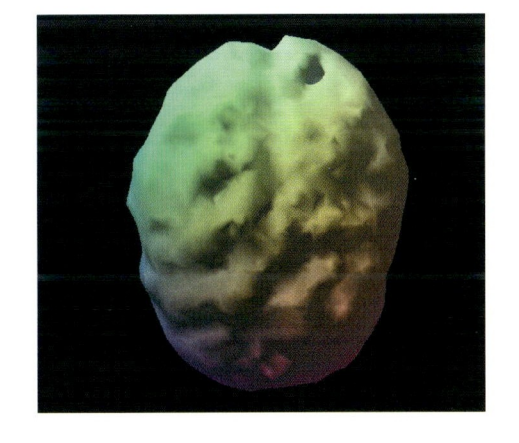

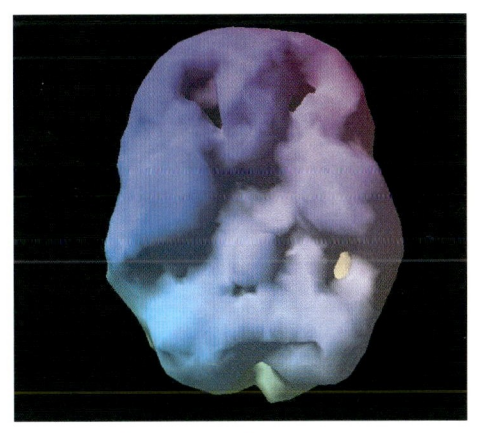

marked overall improvement throughout the cerebral cortex

Section 9

Images of the Ring of Fire

One of the new patterns we feel we have discovered is one we affectionately term the ring of fire. It consists of marked hyperactivity throughout the cortex, often in a ring-like pattern. It shows the hyperfrontality pattern (increased cingulate activity with increased left and right lateral prefrontal cortex activity) frequently seen in obsessive compulsive spectrum disorders and hyperactivity in the left and right lateral parietal and temporal lobe regions. We have seen this pattern most frequently in children and teenagers. It reminds us of the patchy increased uptake seen commonly in Bipolar Disorder. We wonder if it represents a functional brain pattern for children and teens who are vulnerable to Bipolar Disorder. The children and teenagers are not in what most clinicians would consider a manic state and their symptoms may or may not cycle. In a group of 70 patients with this pattern the most common symptoms were moodiness, problems shifting attention, oppositional behavior, irritability, temper problems, hypersensitivity to noise and/or touch, inattention, distractibility and impulse control problems. This pattern seems to be made worse by psychostimulants and serotonergic agents and better by anticonvulsants, such as Depakote or Neurontin and the new antipsychotics, such as Risperdal or Zyprexa.

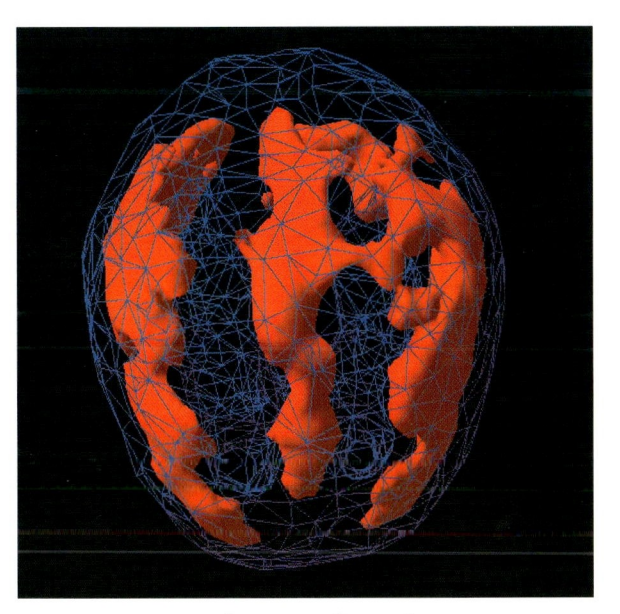

top down surface view

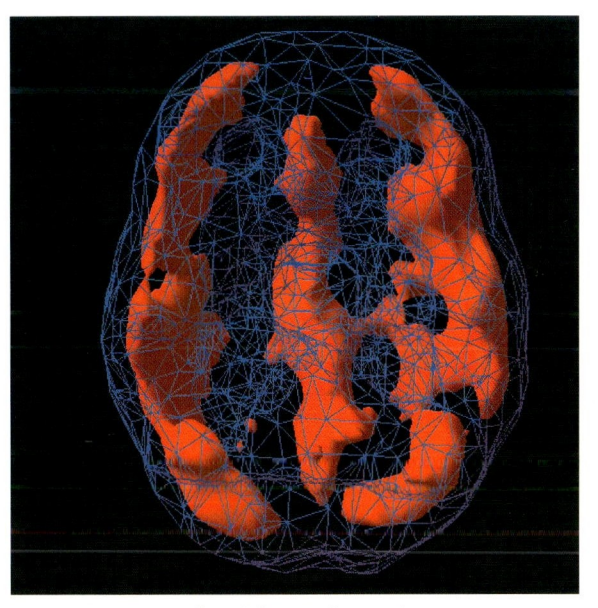

underside surface view

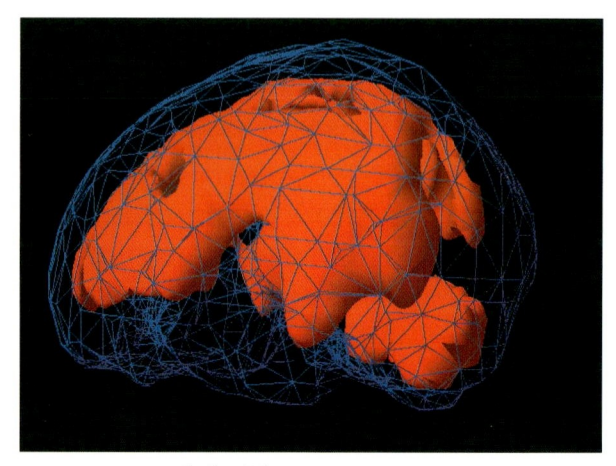

left side active view

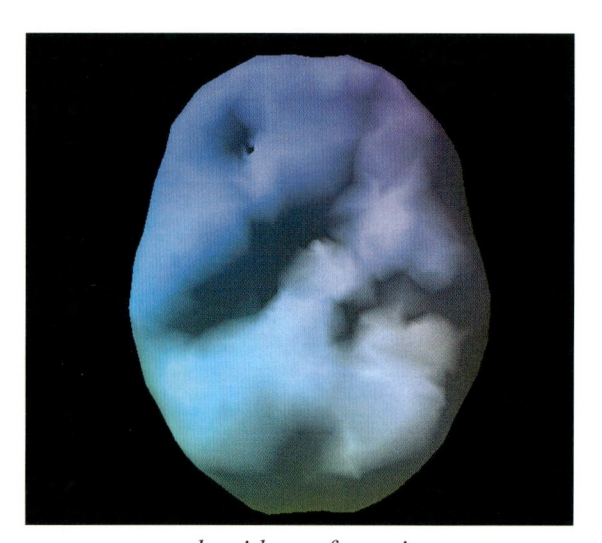

underside surface view 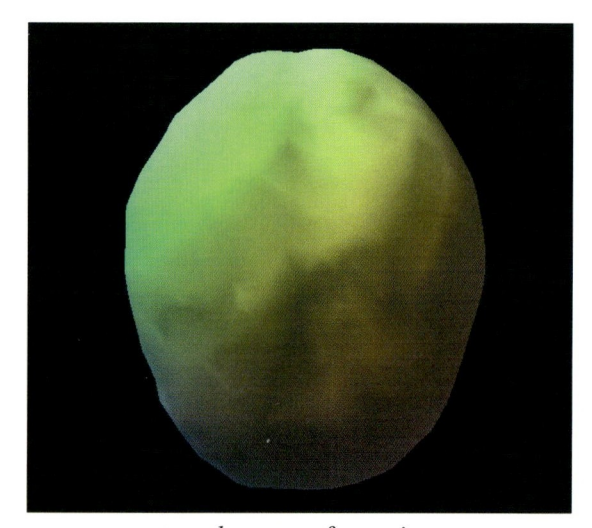   *top down surface view*

Notice the marked hyperactivity throughout the cerebral cortex in a "ring-like" pattern. Also note that the surface views look normal. This scan series is of a 14-year-old boy who had serious problems with oppositional and aggressive behavior. His moods were erratic and he had longstanding behavioral problems despite being a very good student. There was a family history of alcohol abuse and depression. He had a very positive response to Risperdal which had a calming effect on the cerebral hyperactivity.

This next case series is of a 12-year-old girl who was referred to the clinic for aggressive outbursts, moodiness and chronic irritability. Her pattern was similar to the one shown above and she had a similarly positive response to Risperdal.

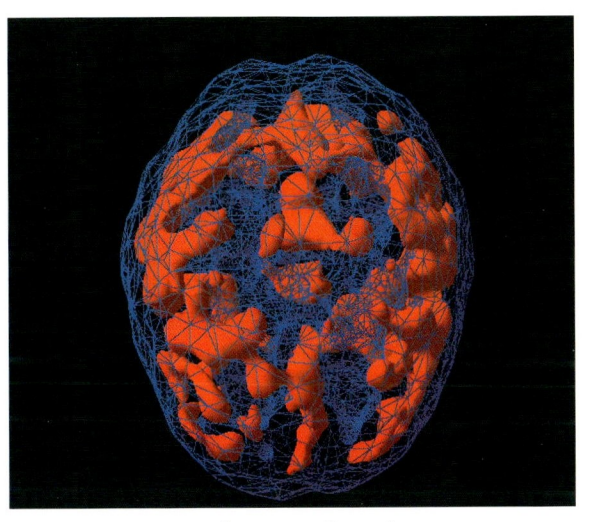

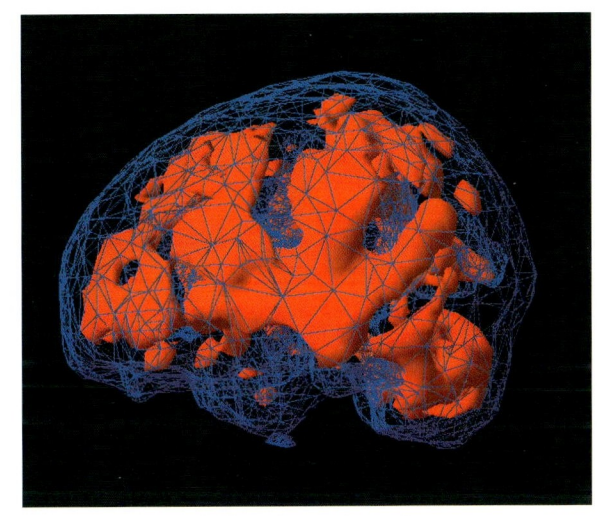

top down active view

left side active view

Tanya, a 17-year-old female, was brought for evaluation because of severe temper problems, conduct problems (runaway and school truancy), a 5-year history of alcohol abuse that had escalated in the prior 2 years and depression with suicidal ideation. Her parents felt her behavior was "willful" and she could change if she wanted to change. Initially they were opposed to psychiatric treatment, but reluctantly came after she had a suicide attempt. Her scan revealed marked hyperactivity throughout the cortex in a "ring of fire" pattern, along with marked increased left basal ganglia activity. She had a nice response to Neurontin and Prozac obtaining more level moods, less temper outbursts and more cooperative behavior.

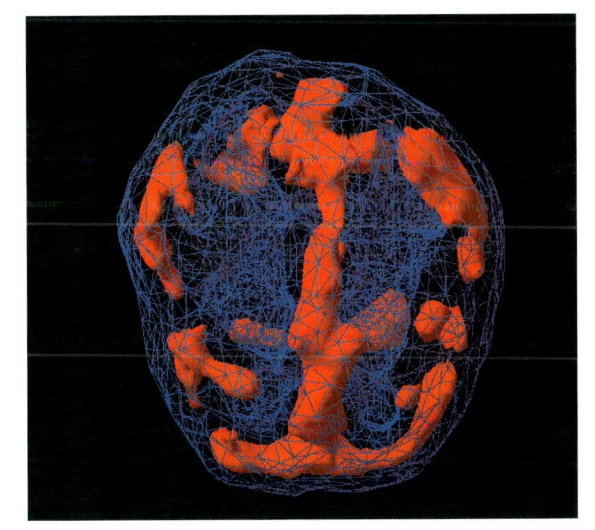

top down active view

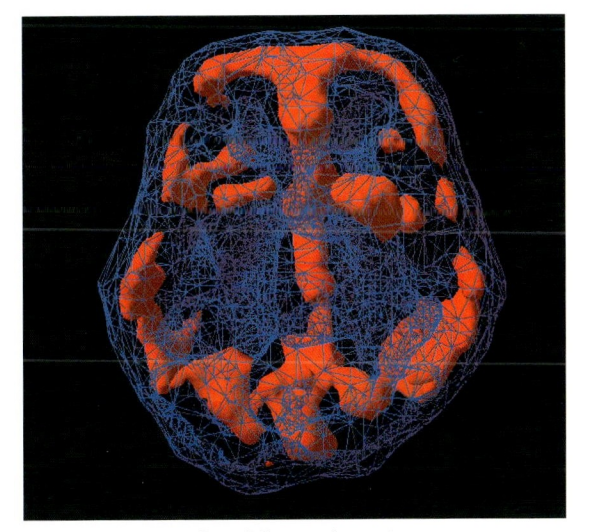

underside active view

The Ring of Fire and Alcohol Induced Violence

A 20-year-old single male, who often became violent when he drank alcohol, even though he reported that alcohol made him feel better. From the age of 18 to 20 he was arrested 10 times for violent, aggressive behavior, all while he was intoxicated. The arrests were mostly for drunk and disorderly in public, one was for assaulting his girlfriend, and the last one, which precipitated the study, was for armed robbery.

On the night of the last crime this man started drinking about 10:00 PM. He drank 750 milliliters of peach schnapps within a half-hour followed by 40 ounces of malt liquor beer the next half-hour. He then "drag raced" a friend on the street and became involved in a motor vehicle accident. He fled the scene on foot. A short while later he called a taxicab. He had the cab driver drive him and a friend around for about 20 minutes. At exactly 12:10 AM he pointed a loaded gun at the cab driver's head and demanded all his money. He got $25 and ran away on foot. The next morning, after sobering up, he turned himself into the police.

At the request of his defense attorney SPECT imaging was performed. Since he seemed to only be aggressive when he drank alcohol he was imaged with and without alcohol. The first SPECT study was performed "drug and alcohol" free. The second study was performed after he consumed 750 milliliters of peach schnapps, followed by 40 ounces of malt liquor beer (the alcohol was the same brand he drank on the night of the crime consumed in the same time frame).

The "non-alcohol" study revealed marked overactivity in the cingulate gyrus, right and left frontal lobes, right and left parietal lobes and the right temporal lobe - the "ring of fire." As noted, these findings are often associated with anxiety, cyclic mood tendencies and irritability.

For the alcohol study, his blood alcohol level was 0.2g/dl(%). This study showed an overall dampening effect on the hyperactive areas of the brain (frontal, parietal and right temporal lobe), with only the cingulate gyrus showing excessive activity (although significantly less activity than on the non-alcohol study). In addition, the right and left prefrontal cortex was now significantly underactive, as were the left and right temporal lobes.

Given the marked hyperactivity in his brain in a drug and alcohol free state, along with his report that he felt more relaxed when he drank, it is not unreasonable to assume he may have been using alcohol as a way to settle down his brain and feel more comfortable (self-medication). Unfortunately, by self-medicating, he was inducing a "violent" pattern in his brain. Increased cingulate activity, abnormal left temporal lobe activity and decreased prefrontal cortex activity is the triad of symptoms that have been found in violent patients. He drank himself into a violent state as a way to medicate underlying abnormalities in his brain.

No Alcohol

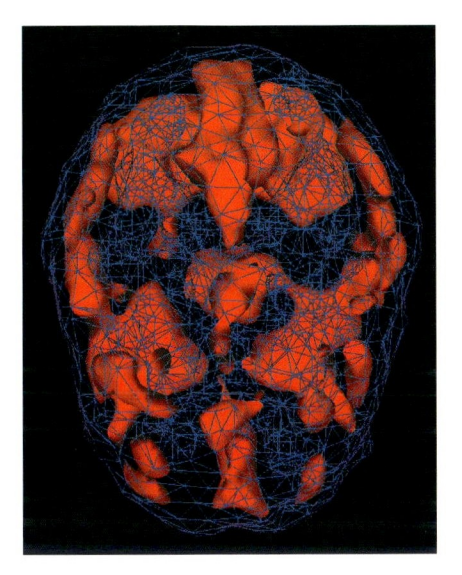

top-down active view
ring of fire pattern

Alcohol Intoxicated State

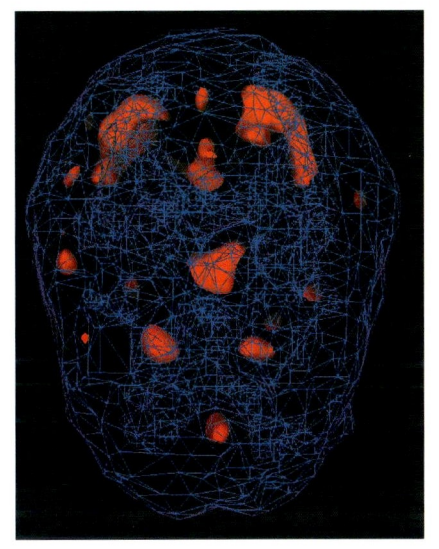

top-down active view
overall dampening effect on the brain
still increased cingulate activity

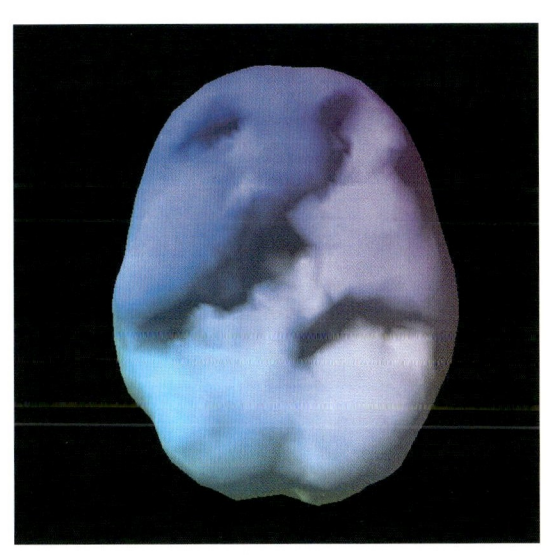

underside surface view
good overall activity without alcohol

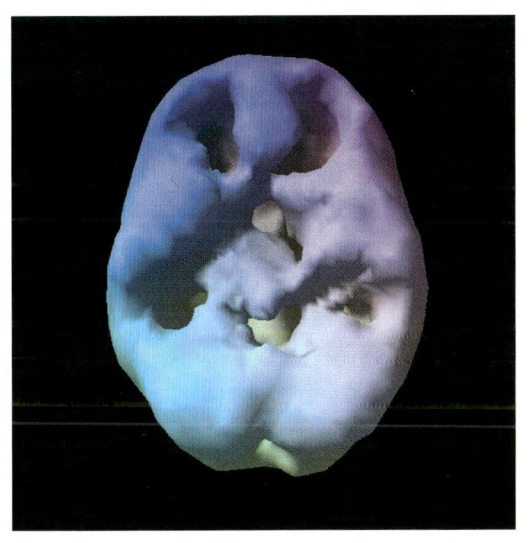

underside surface view
marked decreased in temporal lobes
(tendencies toward aggression),
marked decreased prefrontal cortex
(no internal supervision)

Images of the Ring of Fire

Section 10

Images of PMS

Is it Real? You Bet!

Over the past years we have scanned many women with PMS just before the onset period, during the worst time of their cycle, and then again a week after the onset of their period, during the best time. Most often when PMS is present we see dramatic differences between the scans. When a woman feels good, her deep limbic system is calm and cool and she has good activity in her temporal lobes and prefrontal cortex. Right before her period, when she feels the worst, her deep limbic system is often overactive and she has poor activity in her temporal lobes and prefrontal cortex!

I have seen two PMS patterns, clinically and on SPECT, that respond to different treatments. One pattern is focal increased deep limbic activity often accompanied by temporal lobe hypoperfusion that correlates with cyclic mood changes. When the limbic system is more active on the left side it is often associated with anger, irritability and expressed negative emotion. When it is more active on the right side it is often associated with sadness, emotional withdrawal, anxiety and repressed negative emotion. Left-sided abnormalities are more a problem for other people (outwardly directed anger and irritability), while right-sided overactivity is more an internal problem. Focal deep limbic and temporal lobe findings, worse during the premenstrual period, often respond best to lithium or anticonvulsant medications, such as Depakote, Neurontin, Lamictal or Tegretol. These medications tend to even out moods, calm inner tension, decrease irritability and help people feel more comfortable in their own skin.

The second PMS pattern that I have seen is increased deep limbic activity in conjunction with increased cingulate gyrus activity. The anterior cingulate, as we will see, is the part of the brain associated with shifting attention. Women with this pattern often complain of increased sadness, worrying, repetitive negative thoughts and verbalizations (nagging) and cognitive inflexibility. This pattern usually responds much better to medications that enhance serotonin availability in the brain, such as Zoloft, Paxil or Prozac. Here are several examples.

Haley

Haley is a 12-year-old girl who presented to the clinic with violent mood swings, aggressive behavior, prolonged tantrums, depression and oppositional behavior. Her symptoms primarily occur several days before and after the onset of her menstrual cycle. By the first week after the start of her period she is markedly improved, more compliant, more positive and easier to get along with. In order to help understand the underlying physiological abnormalities in her brain a SPECT series was performed during the worst time of her cycle (day 2 of her menstrual cycle) and during the best time of her cycle (day 10).

Haley's study during the worse part of her cycle was very abnormal with marked overactivity of the anterior cingulate gyrus (associated with obsessive thinking and problems shifting attention), significant decreased temporal lobe activity (associated with aggressive thoughts, hypersensitivity to others, memory problems and mood instability) and marked decreased prefrontal cortex activity (associated with problems of impulsivity, attention span and self-supervision).

The SPECT study during the best time of her cycle markedly improved with decreased anterior cingulate activity and improved function in the temporal lobes and prefrontal cortex. Haley had a positive response to medication geared toward stabilizing the temporal lobes (Neurontin), calming anterior cingulate hyperactivity (Zoloft) and enhancing prefrontal cortex function (Adderall). During the worst time of her cycle she also takes Risperdal to calm the aggressive behavior.

Day 2 of Cycle
During Worst Time

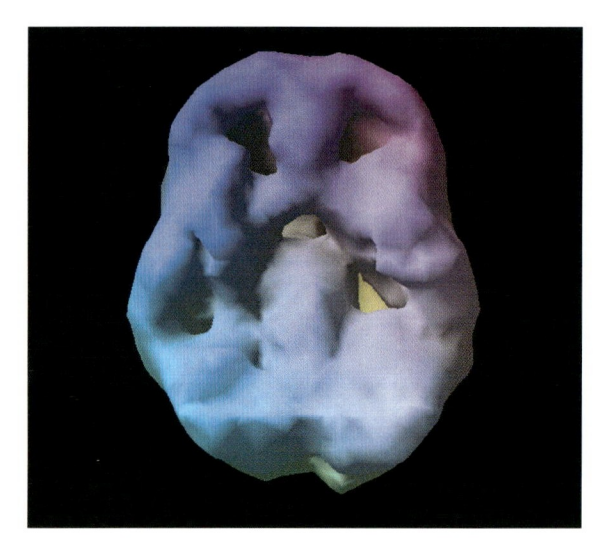

underside surface view
notice marked decreased prefrontal
cortex and temporal lobe activity

Day 10 of Cycle
During Best Time

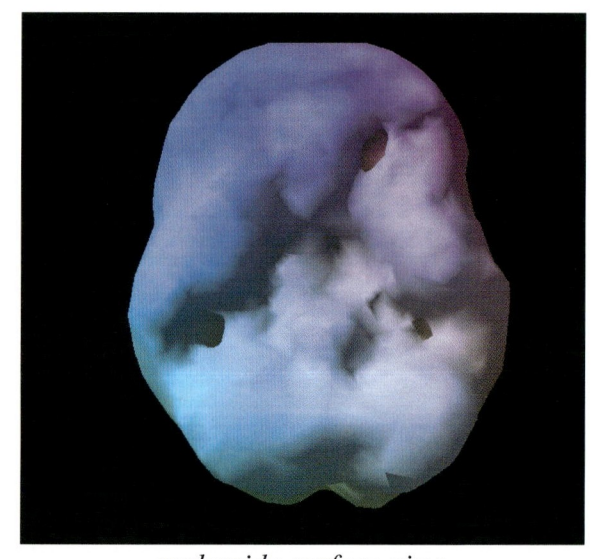

underside surface view
notice marked overall improvement

IMAGES OF HUMAN BEHAVIOR

During Worst Time

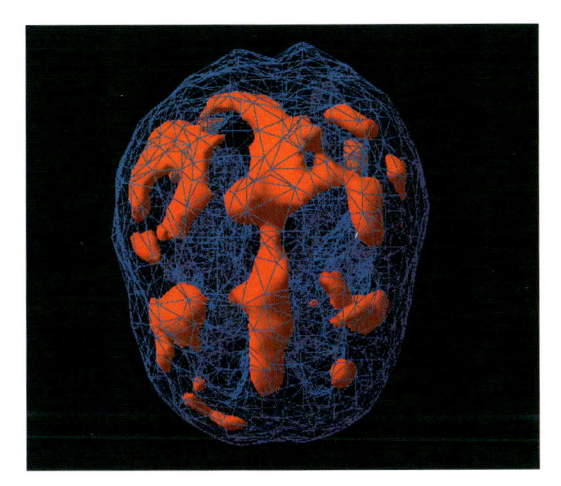

top down active view

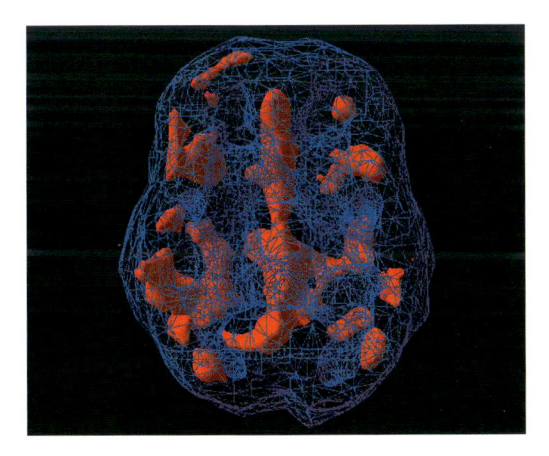

underside active view

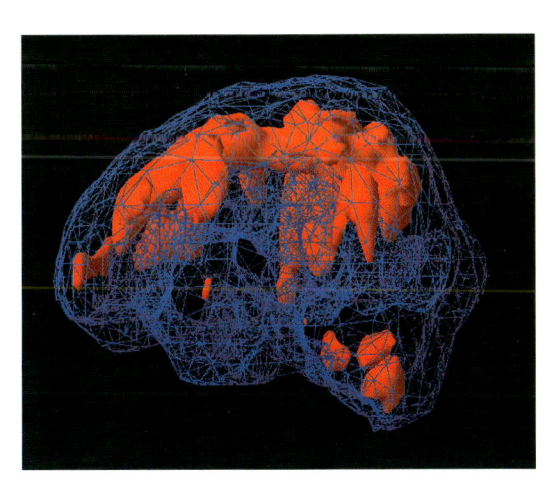

side active view
notice marked increased anterior cingulate activity

During Best Time

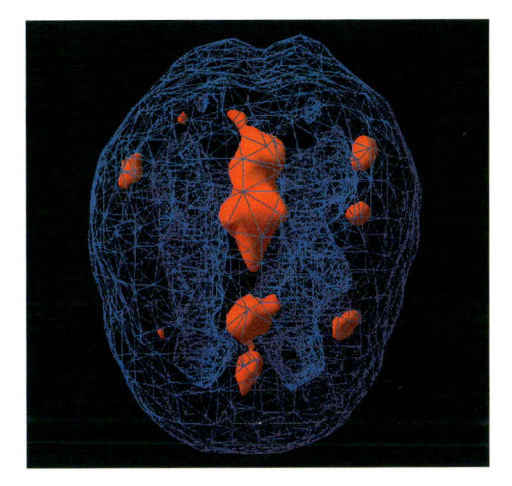

top down active view

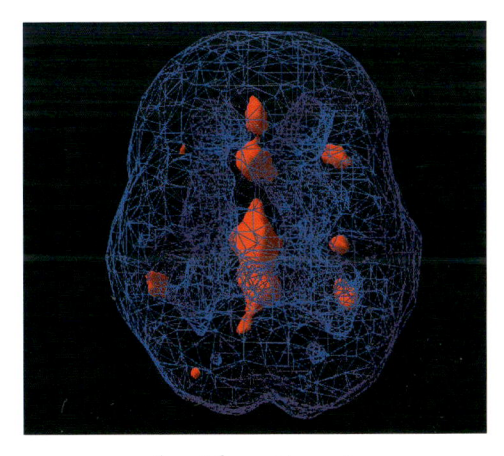

underside active view

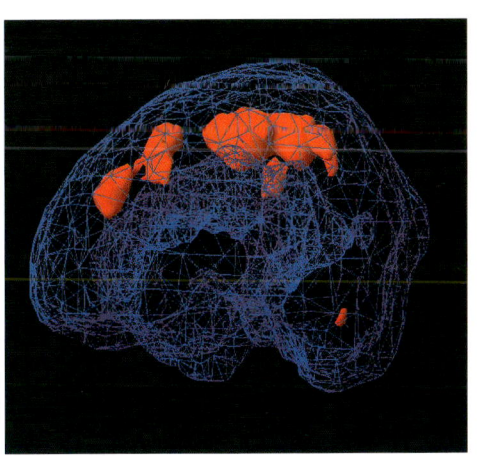

side active view
notice calming of anterior cingulate hyperactivity

Images of PMS

Andrea

Andrea is a 25-year-old female who has been diagnosed with severe PMS and ADD. Seven to ten days before the onset of her menstrual cycle she experiences moodiness, irritability, hypersensitivity to others, anxiety and increased alcohol consumption. These symptoms decrease significantly several days after the onset of her menstrual period.

Just Before Period During Worst Time

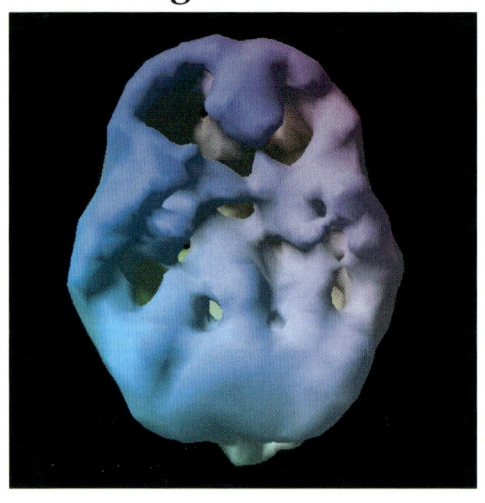

underside surface view
marked decreased prefrontal and temporal activity

top down surface view
notice decreased prefrontal activity

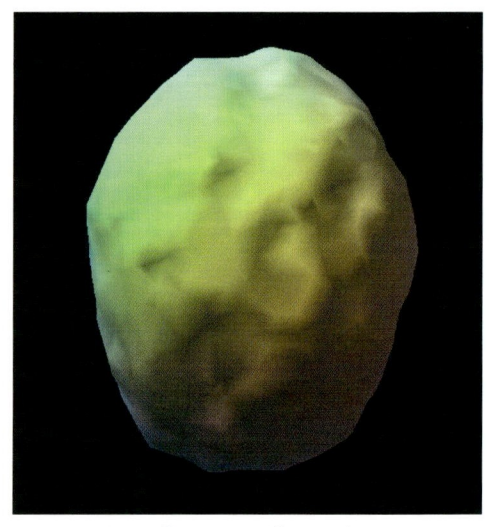

One Week After Period During Best Time

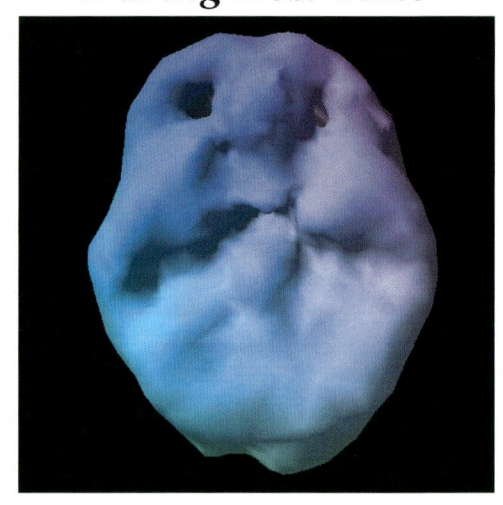

underside surface view
notice marked overall improvement

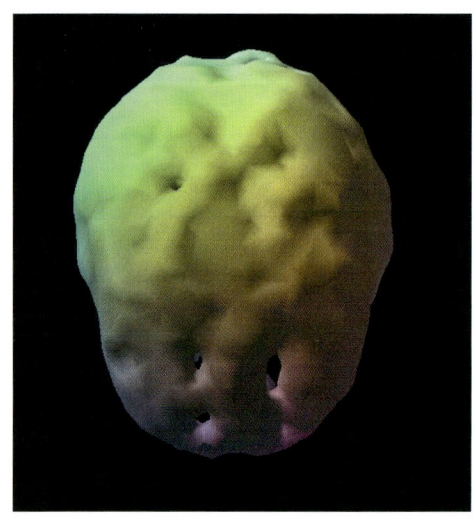

top down surface view
notice fuller prefrontal activity

Images of PMS

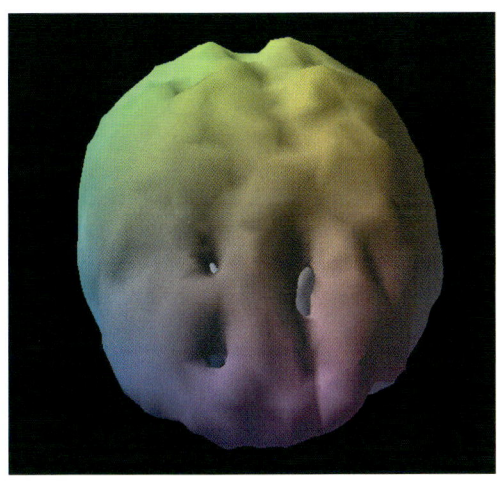

IMAGES OF HUMAN BEHAVIOR

front on surface view
notice decreased prefrontal activity

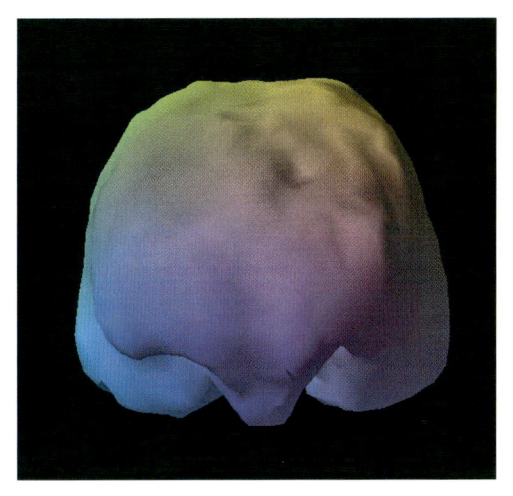

front on surface view
notice fuller prefrontal activity

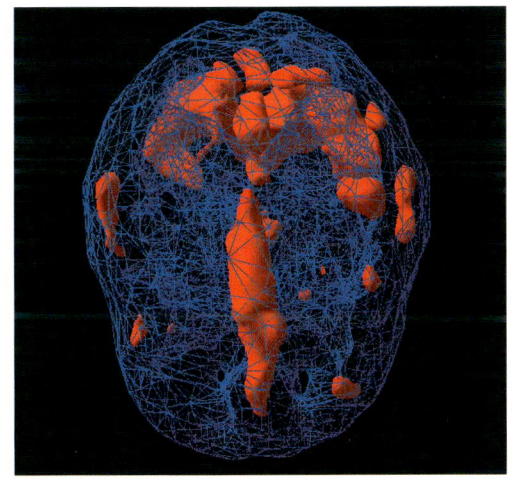

top down active view notice marked increased anterior cingulate activity

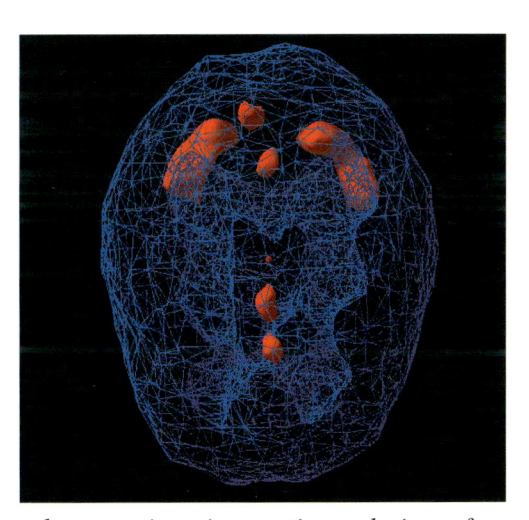

top down active view notice calming of anterior cingulated hyperactivity

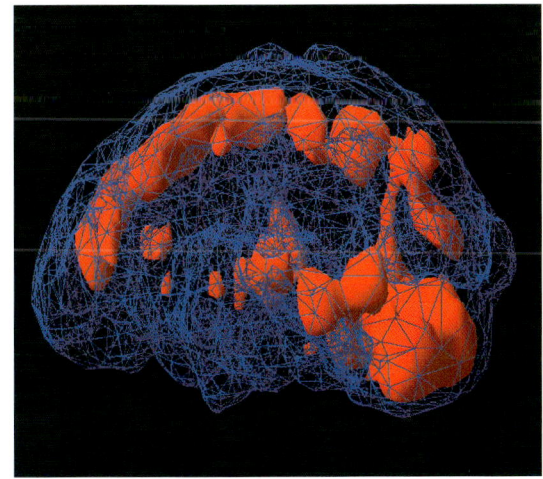

side active view notice marked increased anterior cingulate activity

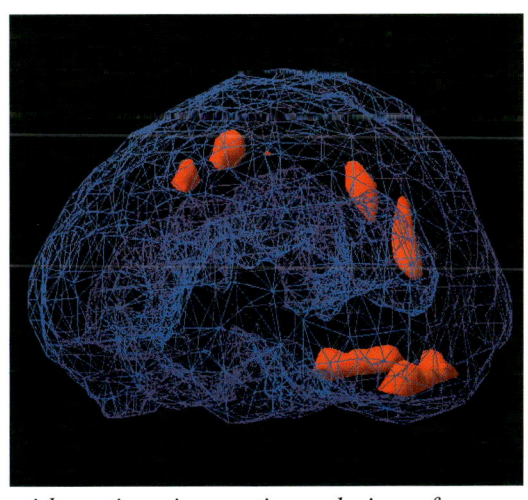

side active view notice calming of anterior cingulate hyperactivity

Images of PMS

Michelle

On three separate occasions Michelle, a 35-year-old nurse, left her husband. Each time she left him it happened within the ten days before the onset of her menstrual period. The last time she left him, her irritability, anger and irrational behavior escalated to the point where she attacked him with a knife over a minor disagreement. The next morning, her husband was on the phone to my office. When I first met Michelle, it was several days after her menstrual period had started and things had significantly settled down. The severe temper outbursts were usually over by the third day after her period started. In my office she appeared to be a gentle, soft-spoken woman. It was hard for me to imagine that this woman had gone after her husband with a carving knife only days before. Because her actions were so serious, I decided to perform two brain SPECT studies on her. The first one was done four days before the onset of her next period – during the roughest time in her cycle – and the second one was done eleven days later – during the best time of her cycle.

My colleagues and I have observed that left-sided brain problems often correspond with a tendency toward significant irritability, even violence. On Michelle's premenstrual brain study before the onset of her period, her limbic system (the mood control center) near the center of her brain was significantly overactive, especially on the left side. This "focal" limbic finding (on one side as opposed to both sides) often correlates with cyclical tendencies toward depression and irritability. There was a dramatic change in her second scan taken eleven days later when Michelle was feeling better. The limbic system was normal!

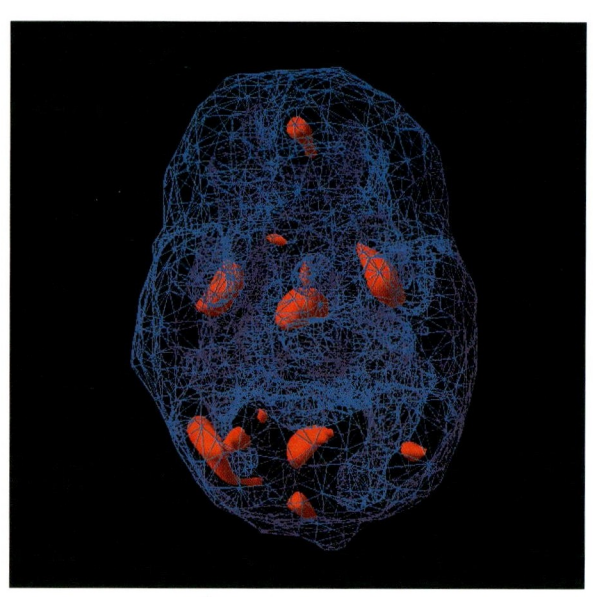

underside active view
notice marked increased limbic activity

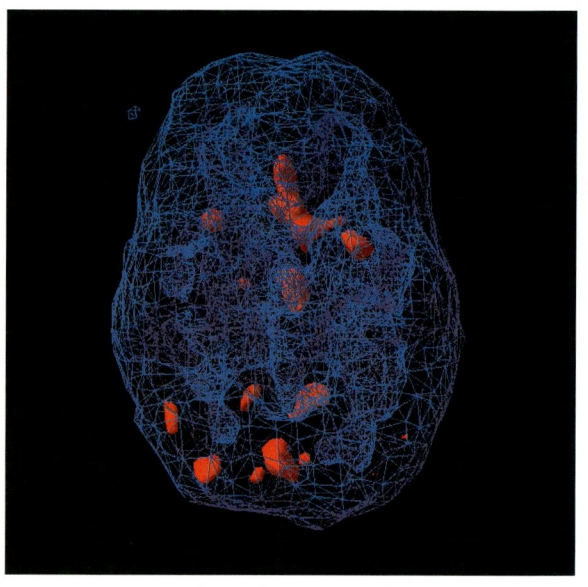

underside active view
notice calming of limbic hyperactivity

JJ

JJ is a 44-year-old woman who experiences severe symptoms before the onset of her period. These symptoms include moodiness, anger, sugar cravings, insomnia and anxiety. These symptoms abate several days after the onset of her period.

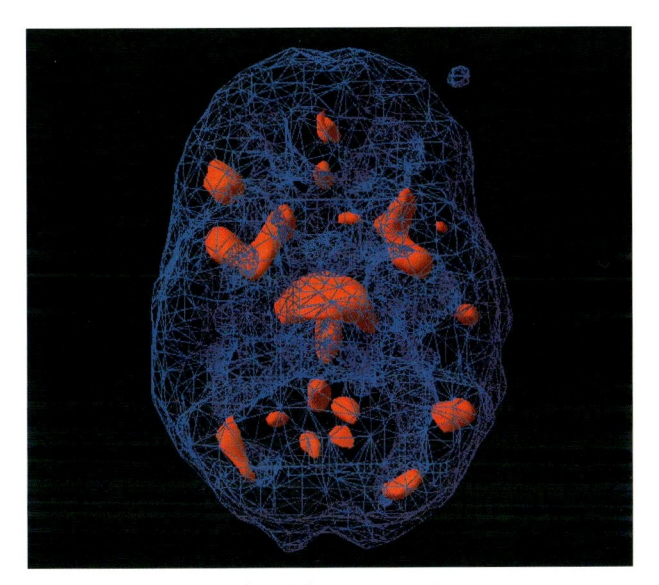

underside active view
notice marked increased limbic activity

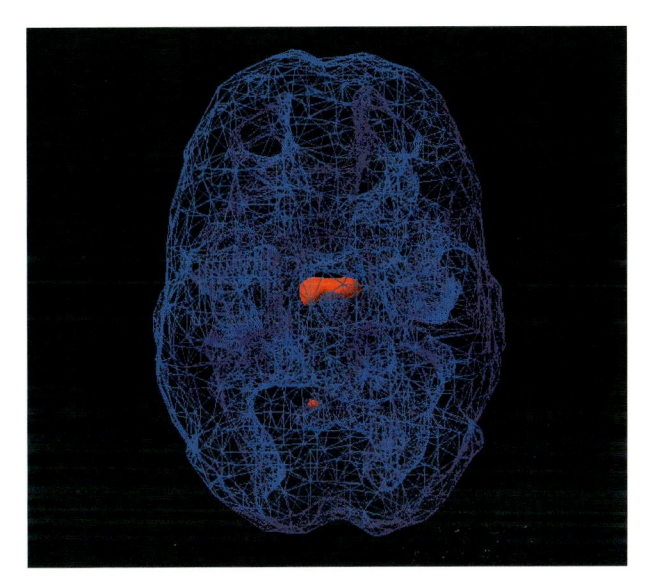

underside active view
notice calming of limbic hyperactivity

Chris

Chris was a thirty-eight-year-old married female referred for evaluation of suicidal thoughts, depression and temper flares. She also experienced problems with anxiety, excessive tension and overeating. These problems occurred primarily during the last 10 days of her menstrual cycle and abated two to three days after the onset of menses. On three separate occassions she left her husband within the 10 days prior to the onset of her period, on one occasion, she attacked him physically. The patient and her husband confirmed the cyclic changes to her symptomatology. Both the patient and her husband kept a symptom log over the next month and she gave consent to participate in the study.

On day 27 (of a 29 day cycle) Chris called the clinic, saying that she was having problems with suicidal thoughts and depression. She was scanned the same day. Her SPECT study revealed significant increased activity in the anterior cingulate gyrus and marked decreased activity in the left temporal lobe and prefrontal cortex bilaterally. She was then scanned on day 8 of the next menstrual cycle when she was symptom free. Her follow-up scan revealed improved temporal lobe and prefrontal cortex function but persistent cingulate hyperactivity.

Due to the clear temporal lobe pathology Chris was placed on divalproate, which stabilized her temper outbursts and suicidal thoughts. Sertraline was then added a month later due to persistent premenstrual sadness. Twenty-four cycles later she remains symptom-free.

Day 27
During Worst Time

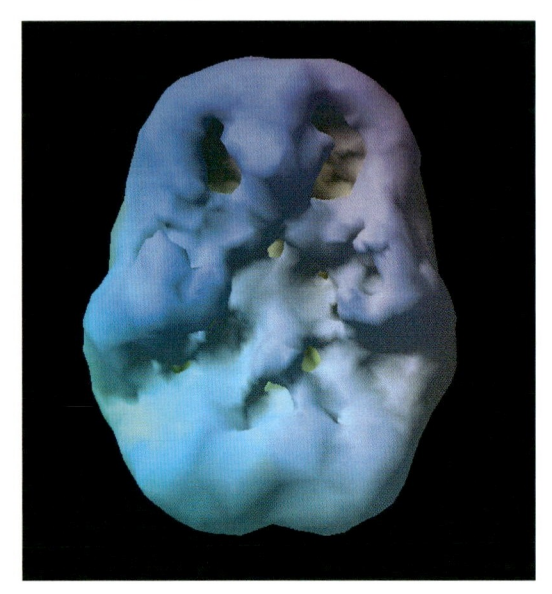

underside surface view
marked decreased prefrontal
and left temporal lobe activity

Day 8
During Best Time

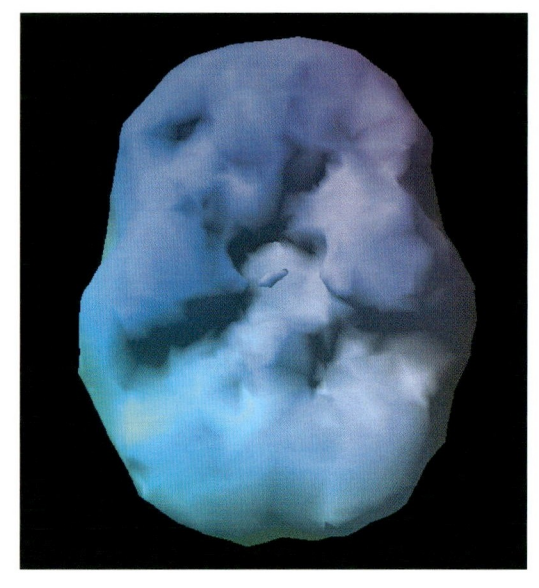

underside surface view
notice marked overall improvement

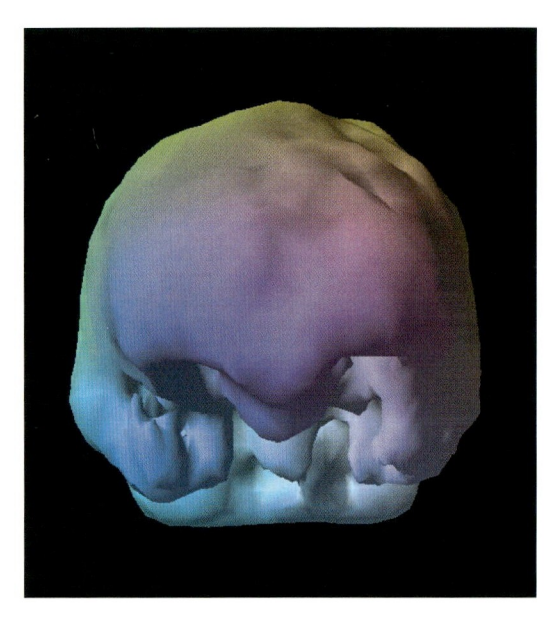

front on surface view
notice decreased prefrontal and
left temporal lobe activity

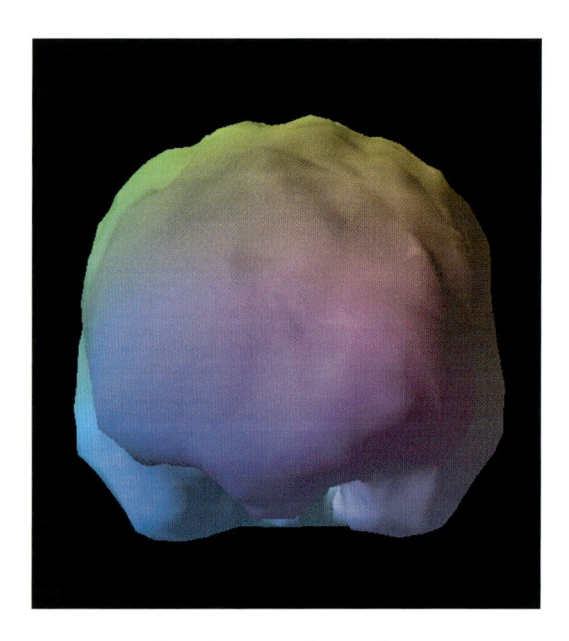

front on surface view
notice fuller prefrontal and
left temporal lobe activity

Images of PMS

IMAGES OF HUMAN BEHAVIOR

Day 27
During Worst Time

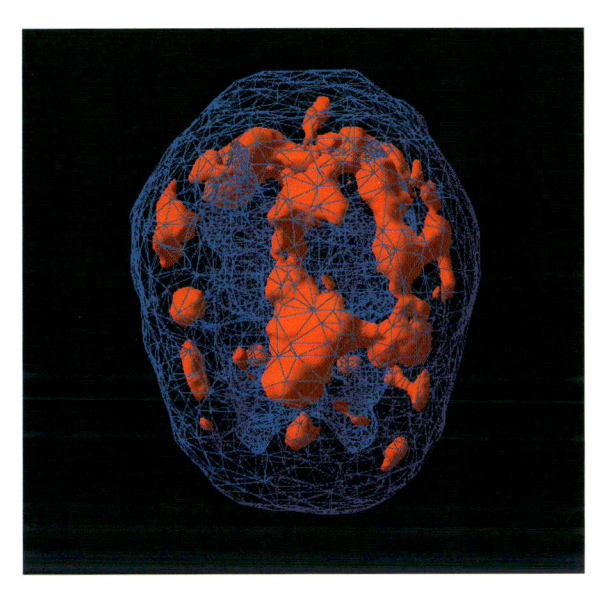

top down active view notice marked increased anterior cingulate activity

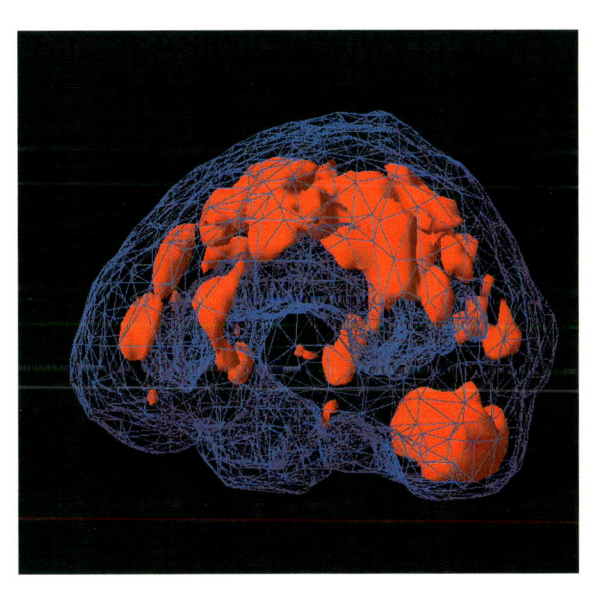

side active view notice marked increased anterior cingulate activity

Day 8
During Best Time

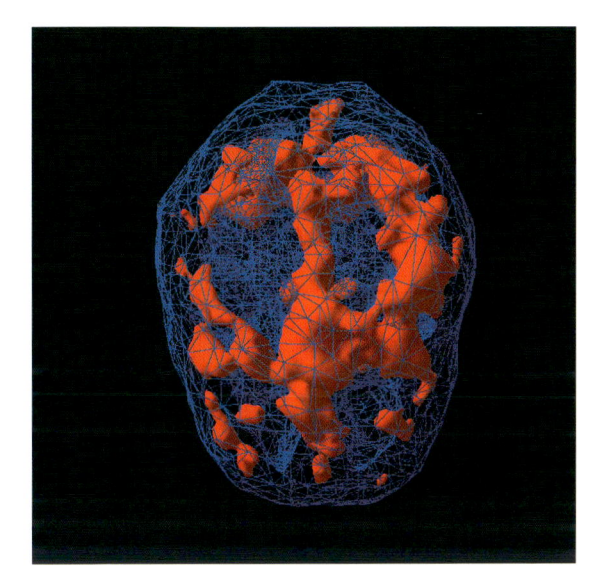

top down active view continued anterior cingulate hyperactivity

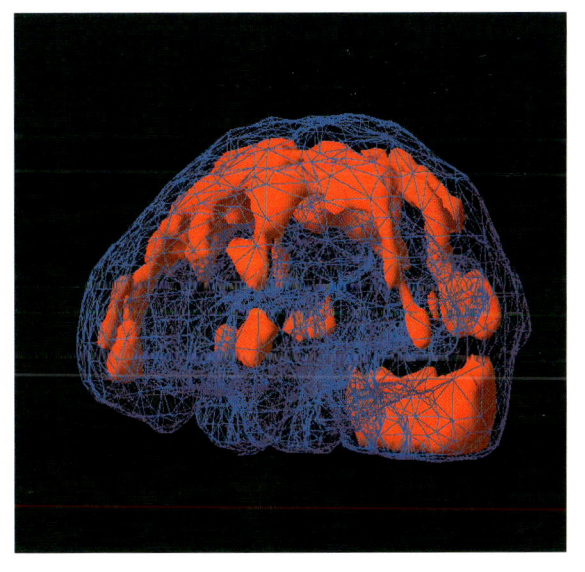

side active view continued anterior cingulate hyperactivity

Images of PMS

Danielle

Danielle was a thirty-three-year-old married female referred for evaluation of suicidal thoughts, depression, anxiety and irritability. These problems occurred predominantly during the last week her menstrual cycle and significantly subsided several days after the onset of menses. She had experienced a post-partum depression after the birth of one child but not after the birth of her other 2 children. The patient and her husband confirmed the cyclic changes to her symptomatology. Both the patient and her husband kept a symptom log over the next month and she gave consent to participate in the study.

On day 25 (of a 28 day cycle) Danielle called the clinic, complaining of severe agitation and moodiness. She was scanned the same day. Her SPECT study revealed significant increased activity in the anterior and central cingulate gyrus and increased activity in the left basal ganglia and deep left temporal lobe. Also, there was decreased activity in the prefrontal cortex and left temporal lobe. She was then scanned on day 10 of the next menstrual cycle when she was symptom-free. Her follow-up scan revealed calming of the cingulate, basal ganglia and temporal lobe hyperactivity and improved activity in the prefrontal cortex and temporal lobes.

Divalproate, sertraline and fluoxetine were ineffective in treating her symptoms, but she had a positive response to lithium carbonate at a dose of 1,200 milligrams a day, with a blood level of 0.6 mcg/dl. Three years later she remains symptom-free during the premenstrual period.

Day 25
During Worst Time

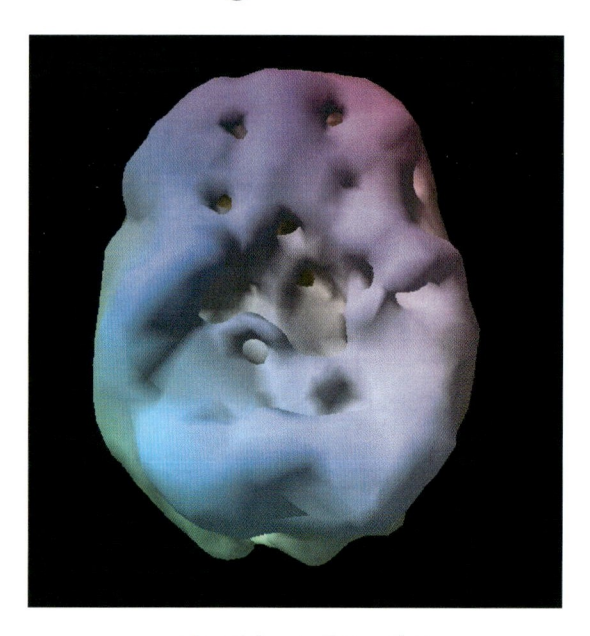

underside surface view
marked decreased prefrontal and temporal activity

Day 10
During Best Time

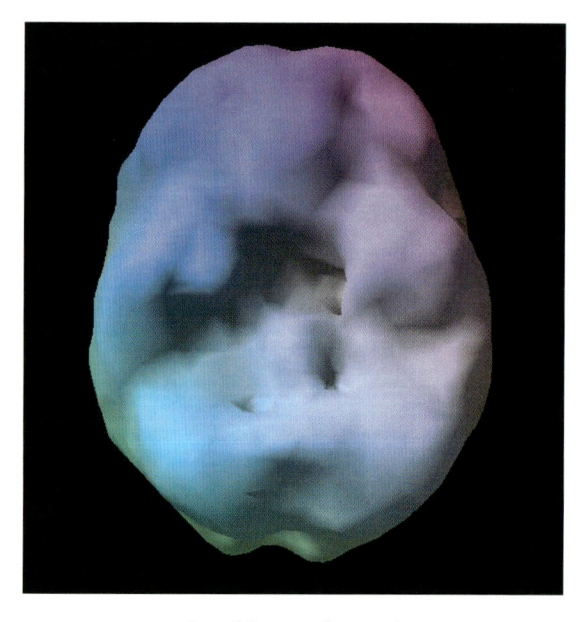

underside surface view
notice marked overall improvement

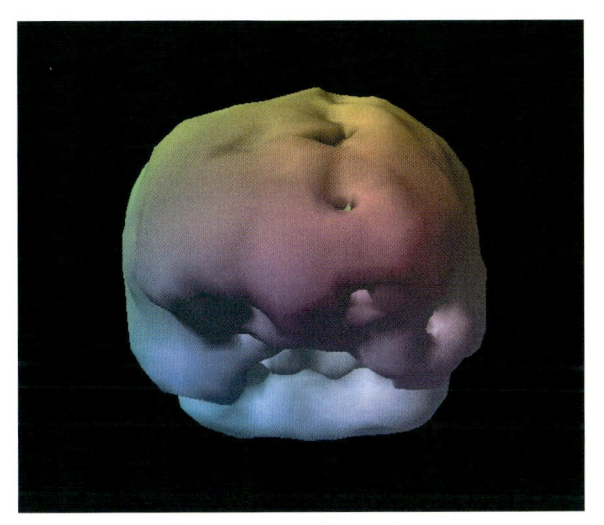

*front on surface view
notice decreased prefrontal and
left temporal lobe (arrow) activity*

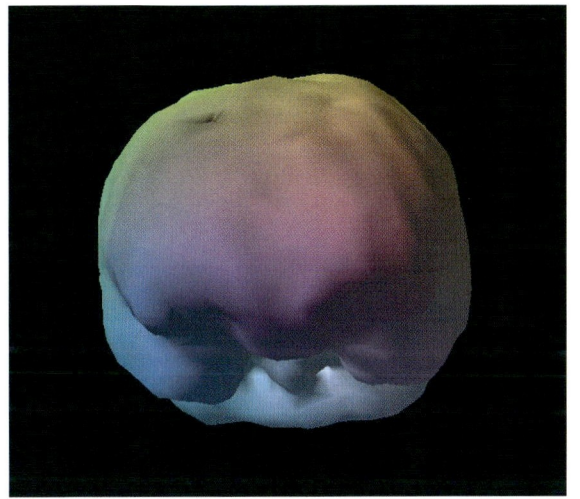

*front on surface view
notice fuller prefrontal and
left temporal lobe (arrow) activity*

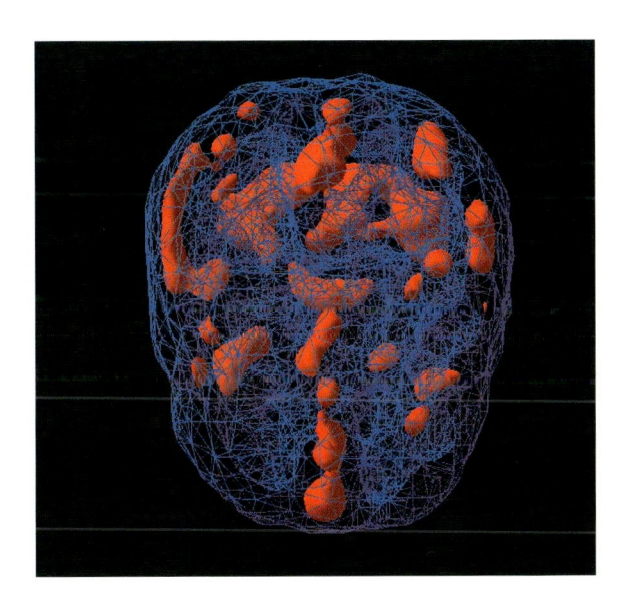

*top down active view notice marked
increased anterior cingulate activity*

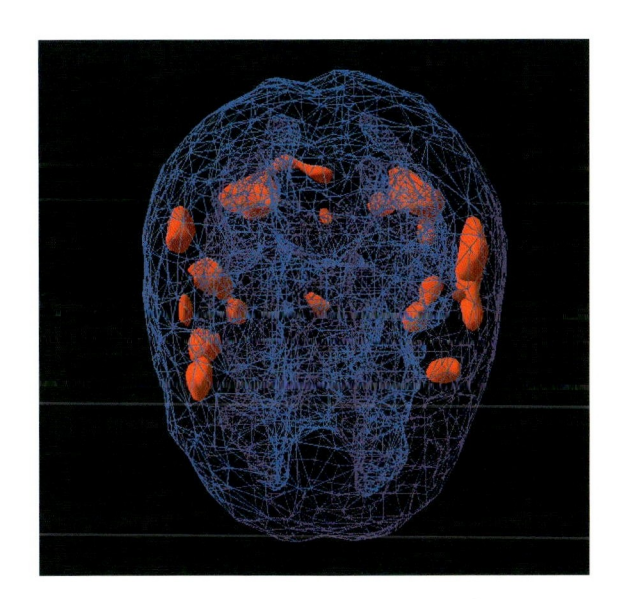

*top down active view notice calming
of anterior cingulate hyperactivity*

Images of PMS

SECTION 11

Images of Anxiety

Increased basal ganglia activity is often a finding we have seen with anxiety disorders. When there is increased activity on the left side it is often associated with anxiety and irritability (expressed anxiety) and when there is increased activity on the right side there is often anxiety, social withdrawal and conflict avoidance. Increased activity in the temporal lobes has also been associated with anxiety. When there is also increased cingulate activity a person may have trouble with repetitive thoughts about his or her anxiety. Here are several examples.

Marsha, a critical care nurse, was forced into treatment by her husband. She was 36-years-old when she first began experiencing panic attacks. She was in a grocery store when all of a sudden she felt dizzy, short of breath, with a racing heart and a terrible sense of impending doom. She left her cart in the store and ran to her car where she cried for over an hour. After her first episode, the panic attacks increased in frequency to the point where she stopped going out of her house, fearing that she'd have an attack and be unable to get help. She stopped working and made her husband take the children to and from school. Her subsequent symptoms typically included shortness of breath, heart palpitations, cold hands, a terrifying sense of impending doom, sweating and negative thinking. She was opposed to any medication, because in the past her mother, in an attempt to treat her own panic attacks, became addicted to Valium and was often quite mean to my patient, Marsha. She did not want to see herself as being in any way like her mother. She believed that she "should" be able to control these attacks. Her husband, seeing her dysfunction only worsen, made the appointment and physically brought her to see a family counselor. The counselor taught her relaxation and how to talk back to negative thoughts, but it didn't help her. Her condition worsened and her husband brought her to see me.

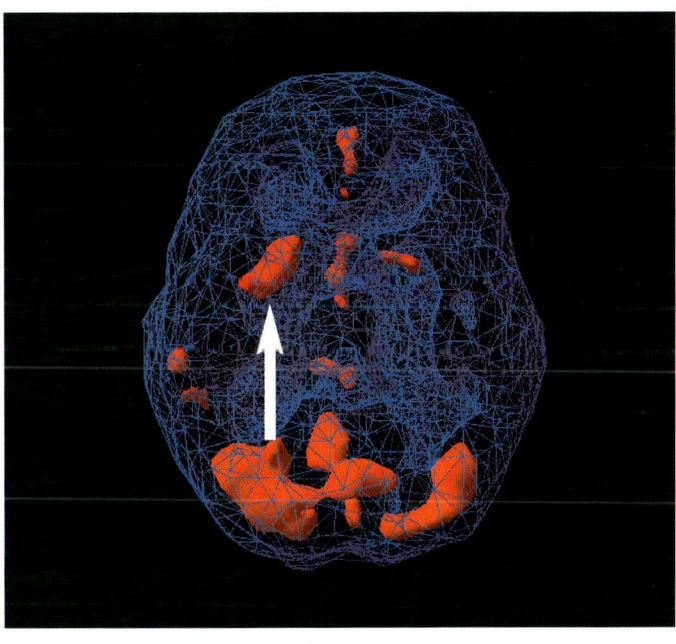

underside active view
note increased right basal ganglia activity (arrow)

Given her resistance to medication I decided to order a SPECT study to evaluate and then also be able to show her her own brain function. Her SPECT study was abnormal. It revealed marked increased focal activity in the right side of her basal ganglia. This is a very common finding in patients who have a panic disorder. Interestingly, patients who have seizure activity also have focal areas of increased activity in their brains. My colleagues and I wonder if the basal ganglia findings are the behavioral equivalent to seizures with the intense level of emotions associated with panic attacks.

The findings on her scan convinced Marsha to try medication. I put her on Klonopin, an anti-anxiety medication that is also used for seizure control. In a short period of time she became able to go out of her house, back to work and resume her life. In addition to the medication, I taught her the group of "Basal Ganglia Prescriptions" (given later) including sophisticated biofeedback and relaxation techniques and worked with her on correcting the negative "fortune-telling" thoughts. Several years later she was able to completely stop her medication and has remained "panic-free."

A Case Of Post Traumatic Stress Disorder

Mark, a 50-year-old business executive, was admitted to the hospital shortly after he tried to kill himself. His wife had just started divorce proceedings against him, and he felt as though his life was falling apart. He was angry, hostile, frustrated, distrusting and chronically anxious. His co-workers felt that he was "mad all the time." He also complained of a constant headache. Mark was also a decorated Vietnam Veteran, an infantry soldier with over 100 kills. He told me that he lost his humanity in Vietnam and that the experience made him "numb."

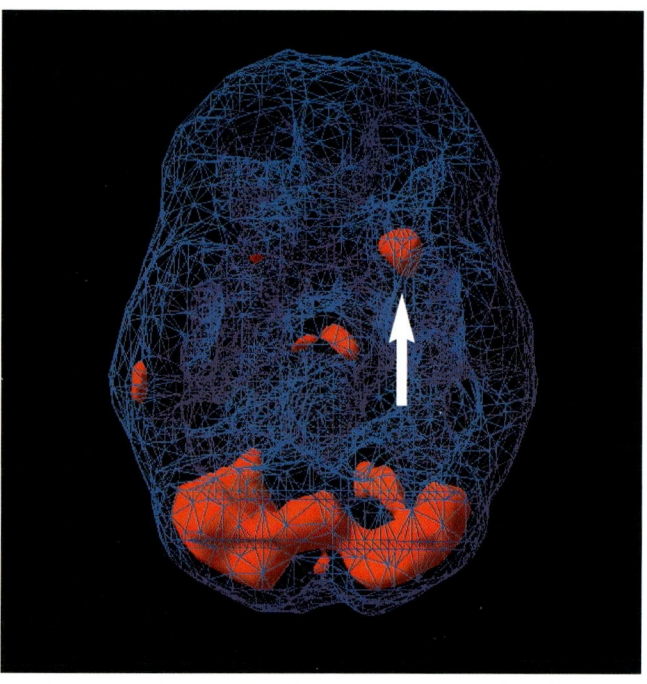

underside active view
note increased left basal ganglia activity (arrow)

In the hospital, he said that he was tormented by the memories of the past. Mark had post traumatic stress disorder (PTSD). He felt that with his wife leaving him, he had no reason to live. Due to the severity of his symptoms, along with a history of a head injury in Vietnam, I ordered a brain SPECT study. It was abnormal, showing marked increased activity in the left basal ganglion. It was the most intense activity in that part of the brain I had ever seen.

Left-sided basal ganglion findings are often seen in people who are chronically irritable or angry. Mood stabilizers, such as Lithium, Tegretol, or Depakote, are often helpful in decreasing the irritability and calming down focal "hot" areas in the brain. I placed Mark on Depakote. Almost immediately, his headaches went away and he began to feel calmer. The hospital staff noted how much calmer he was. He stopped snapping at everyone and he became more able to do the psychological work of healing from his divorce and the wounds from Vietnam.

In working with Mark, I often felt that his experiences in Vietnam had reset his basal ganglia to be constantly on the alert. Nearly everyday for 13 months of the war, he had to be "on alert" in order to avoid being shot. Through the years, he never had the chance to learn how to reset his brain back to normal. The medication and therapy allowed him to relax, and feel, for the first time in 25 years, that he had truly left the war zone.

Here are several other examples.

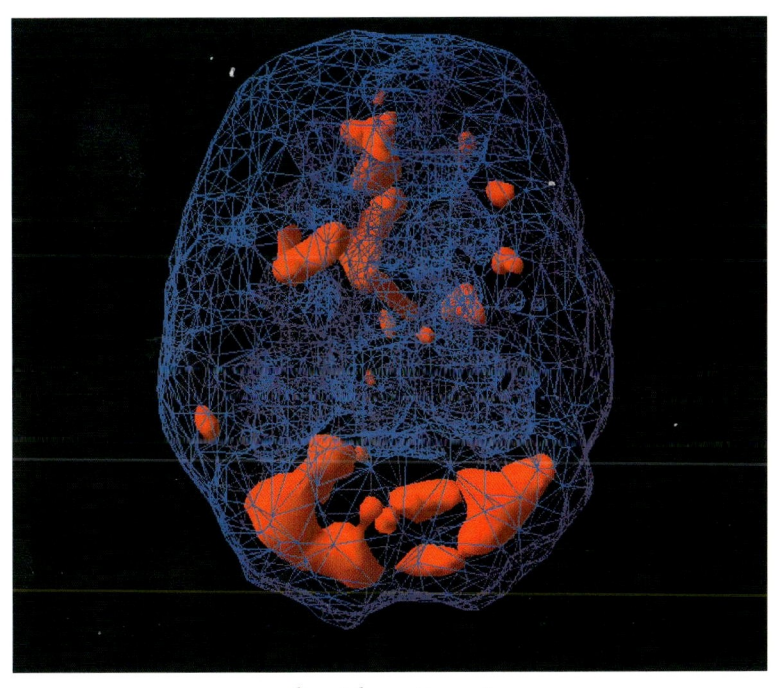

underside active view
note increased right basal ganglia
28 year old woman with chronic anxiety, conflict avoidance

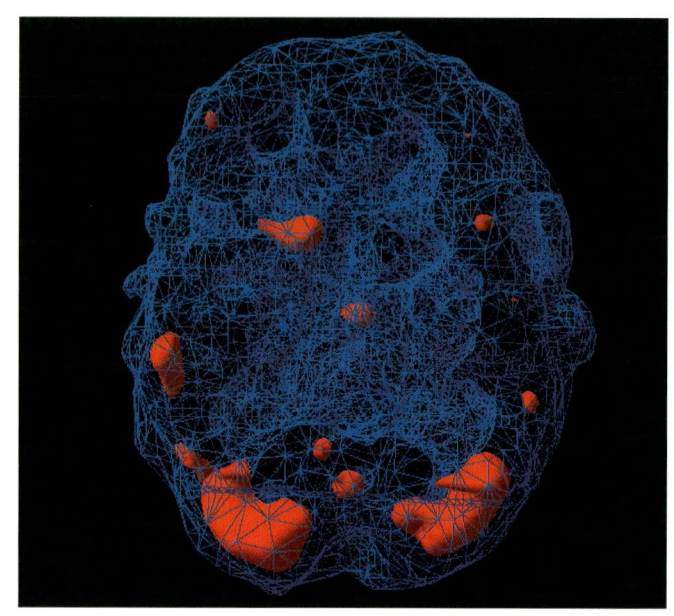

underside active view
note increased right basal ganglia
44-year-old man with chronic mild anxiety, conflict avoidance

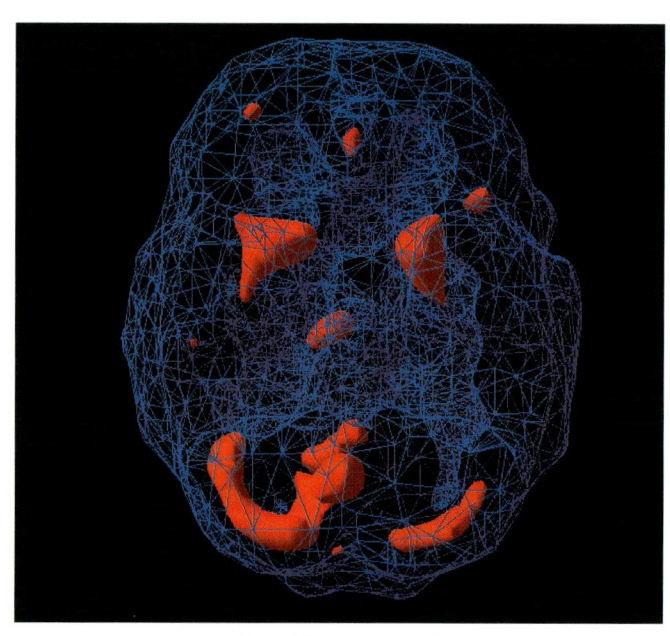

underside active view
note increased right and left basal ganglia
48-year-old man with panic disorder

Section 12

Images of Attention Deficit Disorder

The first evidence of the brain being understimulated in attention deficit disorder was introduced with the use of more advanced electroencephalograms (EEG or brainwave studies) by Joel Lubar from the University of Tennessee. He demonstrated that when ADD children and teenagers performed a concentration task there was an increased amount of slow brain wave activity in their frontal lobes, instead of the usual increase in fast brain wave activity that was seen in the majority of the control group.

In 1990, Alan Zametkin, MD published PET data that supported the notion of brain underactivity in the prefrontal cortex, especially in response to an intellectual challenge. Data from my own work with brain SPECT imaging drew the same conclusions. At rest most ADD people have normal activity in their brain. When they perform a concentration task, however, they experience decreased activity in the prefrontal cortex, rather than the expected increased activity that is seen in a normal control group.

Tied to the decreased prefrontal cortex findings are the studies that indicate that ADD has a large genetic contribution, involving dopamine availability in the brain. A significant amount of dopamine is produced in the basal ganglia (large, structures deep within the brain). Stimulant medications work by enhancing dopamine availability in this part of the brain. Studies have demonstrated that the basal ganglia is smaller in people with ADD. The basal ganglia have a significant number of nerve tracks that go through the limbic system to the prefrontal cortex. It appears that when there is not enough dopamine available in the basal ganglia then there is not enough "fuel" to drive the frontal lobes when they need to activate with concentration.

In addition to the genetic contribution to ADD, maternal alcohol or drug use, birth trauma, jaundice, brain infections and head trauma (sometimes even minor ones, especially to the left prefrontal cortex) can play a causative role.

Subtypes of ADD

It is essential to note that ADD is a developmental disorder diagnosed through clinical history over a prolonged period of time. Brain imaging is not necessary to make the diagnosis of ADD, although it may be helpful in certain complicated cases. Based on my brain imaging experience I have seen 7 clinical subtypes of ADD:

1. AD/HD, combined type with both symptoms of inattention and hyperactivity-impulsivity. Brain SPECT imaging typically shows decreased activity in the basal ganglia and prefrontal cortex during a concentration task. This subtype of ADD typically responds best to psychostimulant medication.

Rest, Concentration & Concentration with Medication

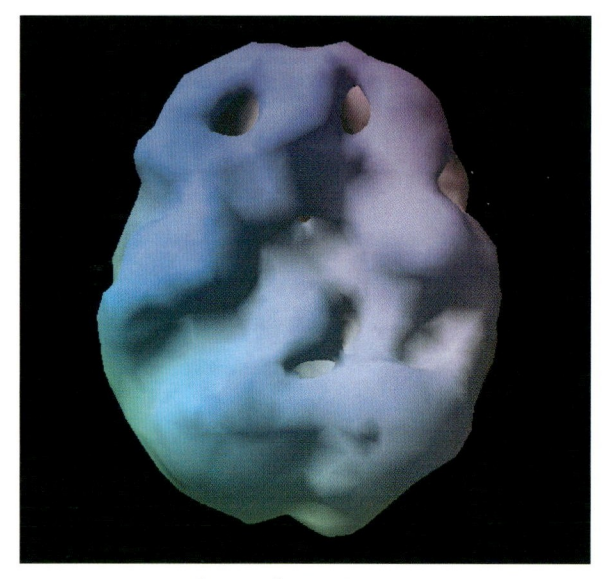

undersurface view, rest
mild decrease prefrontal area

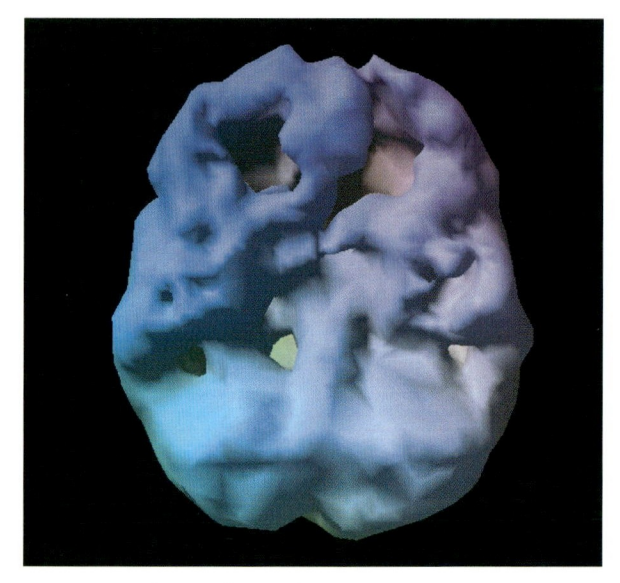

undersurface view, concentration
marked decrease prefrontal cortex and left temporal lobe

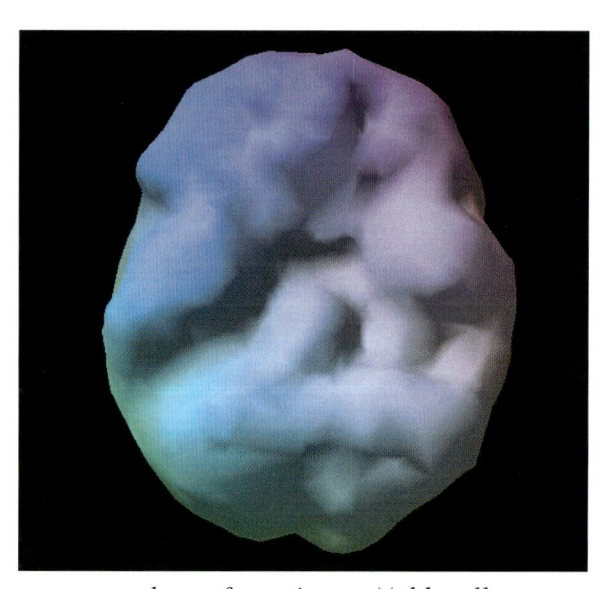

undersurface view, w/Adderall
overall marked improved activity

2. AD/HD, primarily inattentive subtype with symptoms of inattention and also chronic boredom, decreased motivation, internal preoccupation and low energy. Brain SPECT imaging typically shows decreased activity in the basal ganglia and dorsal lateral prefrontal cortex during a concentration task. This subtype of ADD also typically responds best to psychostimulant medication.

Before & After Treatment with Ritalin & Adderall

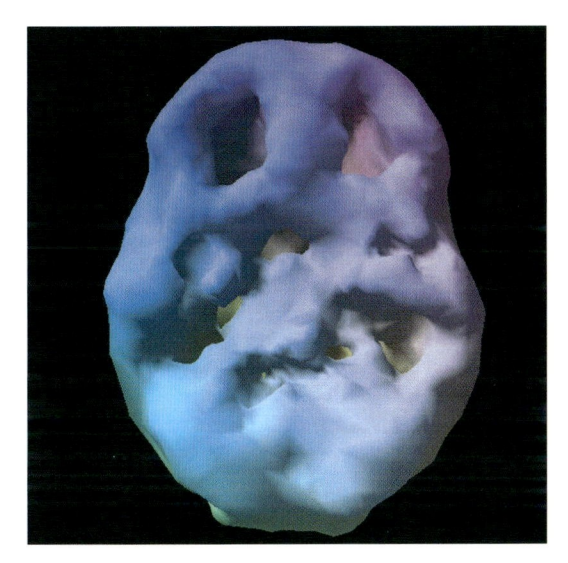

undersurface view, NO MEDS
poor prefrontal and temporal lobe activity

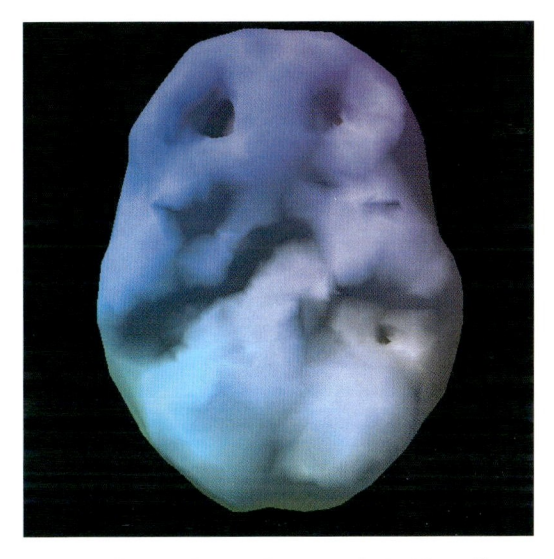

undersurface view, with Adderall
marked overall improvement

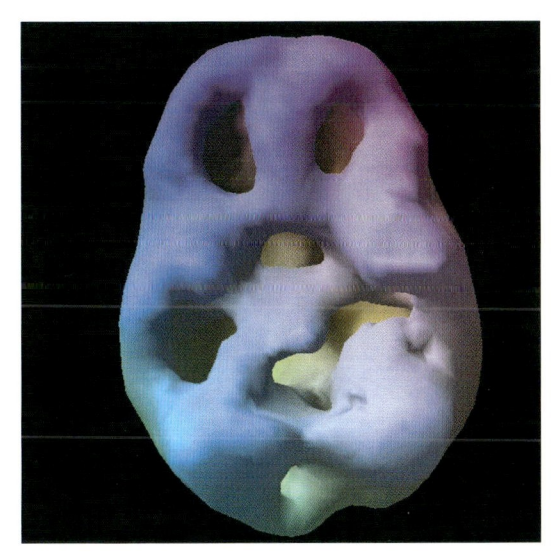

undersurface view, NO MEDS
overall severe decreased activity

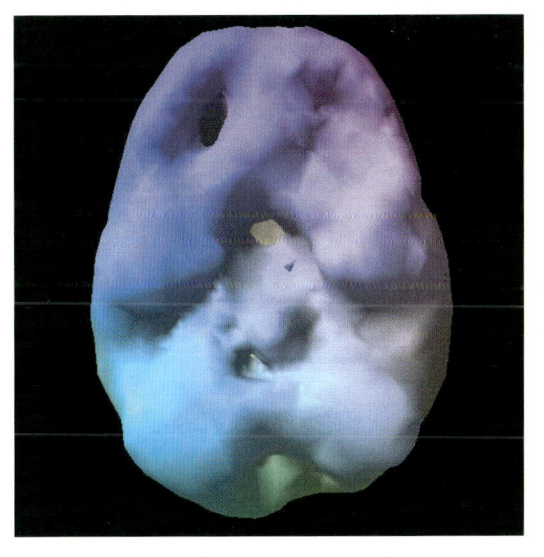

undersurface view, w/Ritalin
overall marked improved activity

3. **Overfocused ADD**, with symptoms of trouble shifting attention, cognitive inflexibility, difficulty with transitions, excessive worrying, and oppositional and argumentative behavior. There are often symptoms of inattention and hyperactivity-impulsivity. Brain SPECT imaging typically shows increased activity in the anterior cingulate gyrus and decreased prefrontal cortex activity. This subtype typically responds best to medications that enhance both serotonin and dopamine availability in the brain, such as venlafaxine or a combination of an SSRI (such as fluoxetine or sertraline) and a psychostimulant.

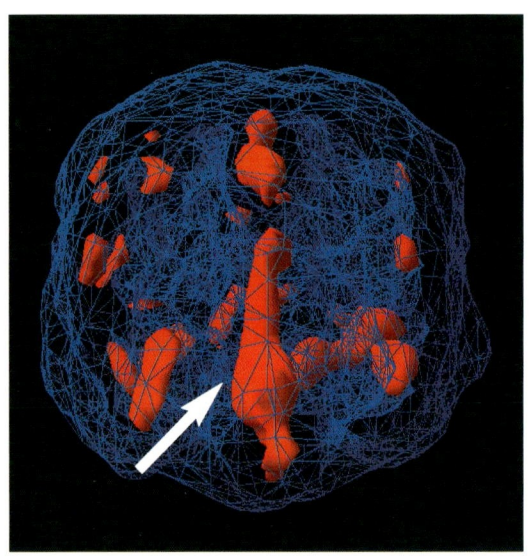

front on active view increased anterior cingulate activity

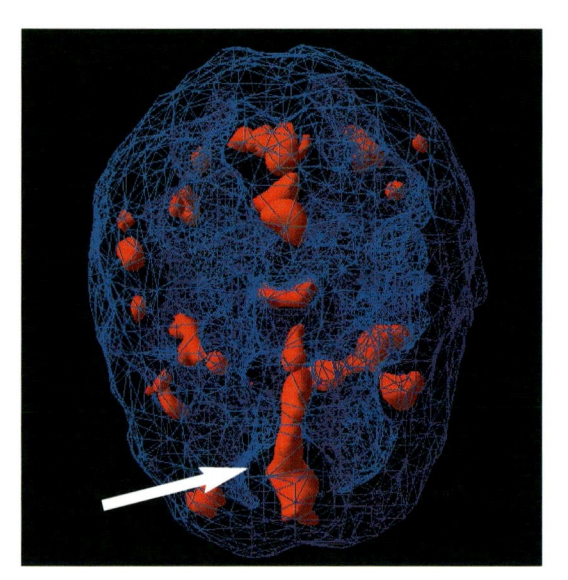

active top down view increased anterior cingulate activity

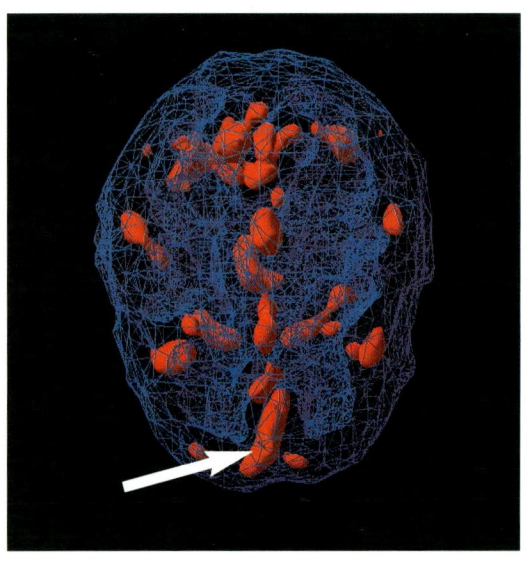

top down active view increased anterior cingulate activity

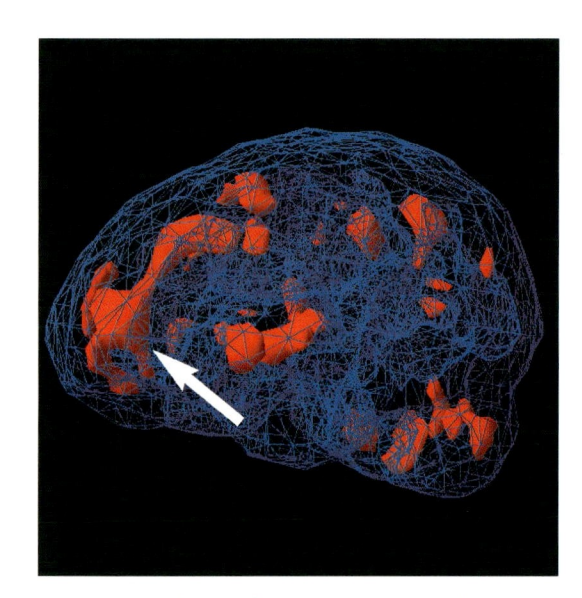

active side view increased anterior cingulate activity

4. Temporal lobe ADD, with symptoms of inattention and/or hyperactivity-impulsivity and mood instability, aggression, mild paranoia, anxiety with little provocation, atypical headaches or abdominal pain, visual or auditory illusions, and learning problems (especially reading and auditory processing). Brain SPECT imaging typically shows decreased or increased activity in the temporal lobes with decreased prefrontal cortex activity. Aggression tends to be more common with left temporal lobe abnormalities. This subtype typically responds best to anticonvulsant medications (such as gabapentin, divalproate, or carbamazepine) and a psychostimulant.

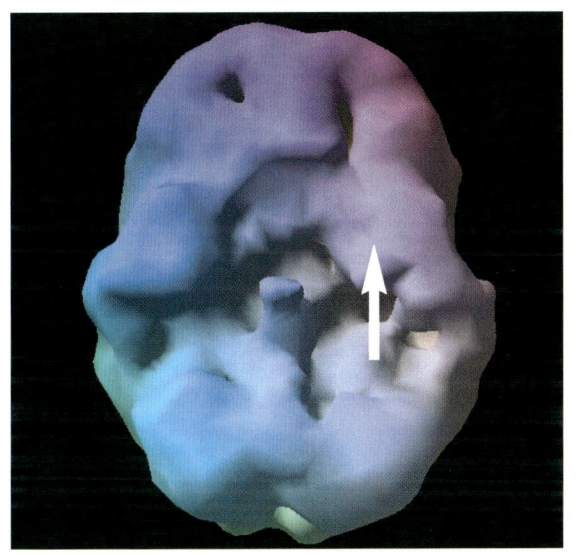

undersurface view
decreased left temporal lobe activity

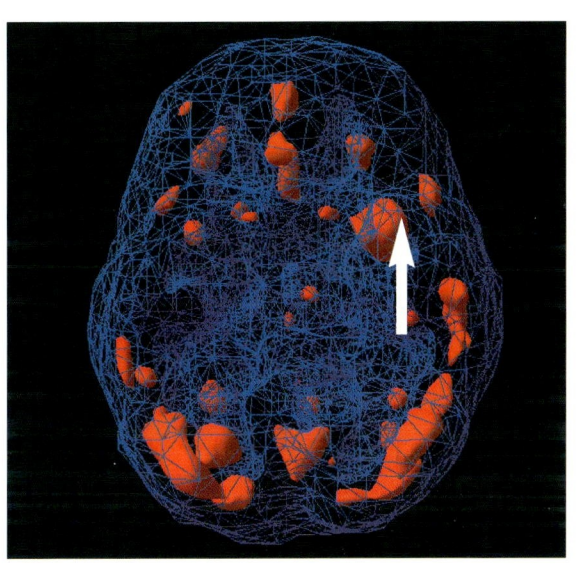

underside active view
increased left temporal lobe activity

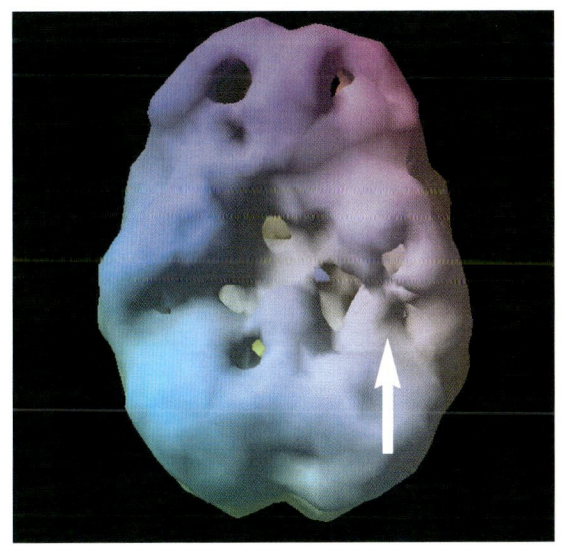

undersurface view
marked decreased left
temporal lobe activity

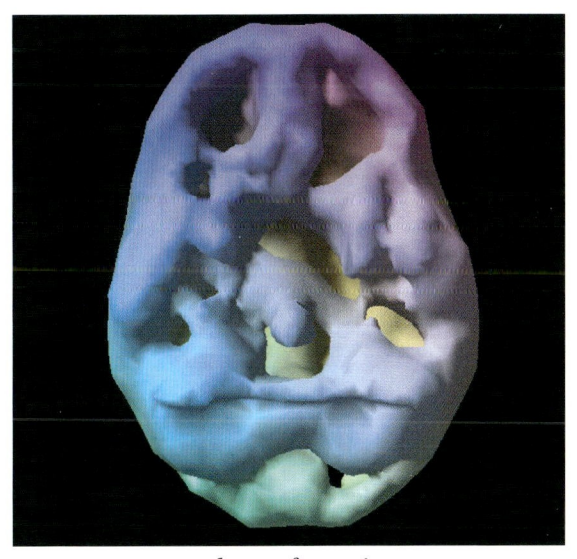

undersurface view
marked decreased temporal
and prefrontal cortex bilaterally

5. Limbic ADD, with symptoms of inattention and/or hyperactivity-impulsivity and negativity, depression, sleep problems, low energy, low self-esteem, social isolation, decreased motivation and irritability. Brain SPECT imaging typically shows increased central limbic system activity and decreased prefrontal cortex activity. This subtype typically responds best to stimulating antidepressants such as buprion or imipramine, or venlafaxine if obsessive symptoms are present.

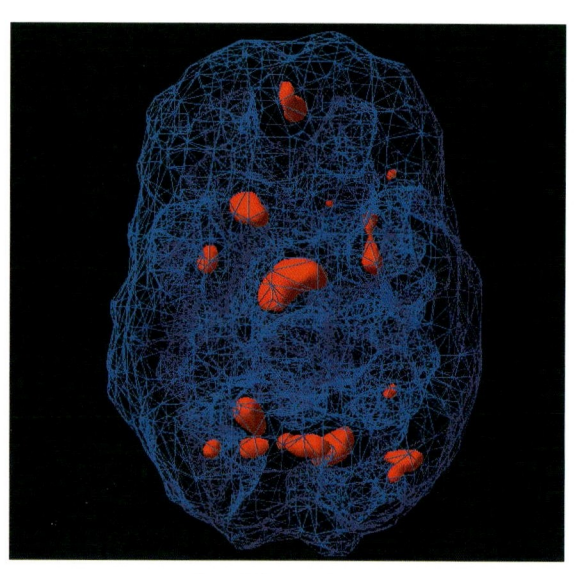

underside active view
increased limbic activity

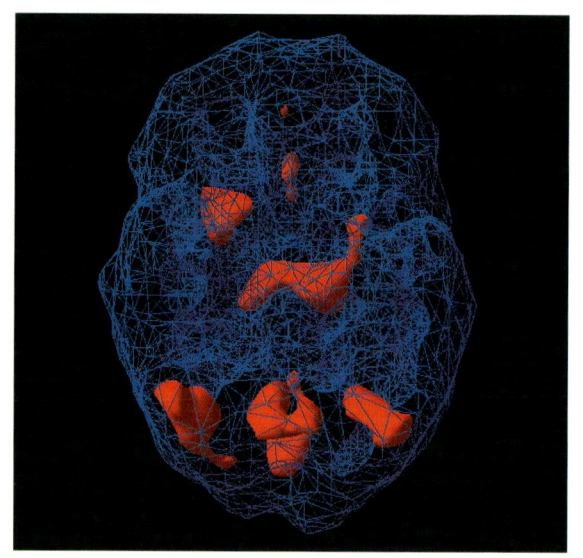

underside active view
increased limbic activity

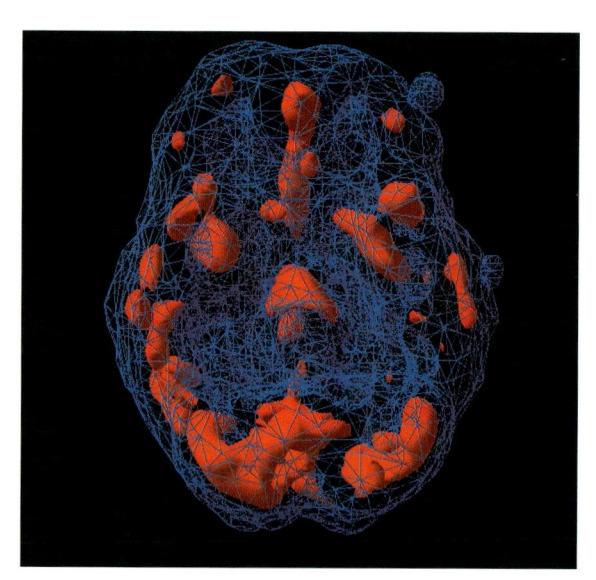

underside active view marked increased limbic,
basal ganglia and anterior cingulate activity

6. **Trauma Induced ADD**, especially to the left dorsolateral prefrontal cortex. The symptoms come on or intensify in the year after a head injury. The ADD symptoms may respond to psychostimulant medication. If irritability results secondary to psychostimulant medication the addition of a low dose anticonvulsant may be helpful.

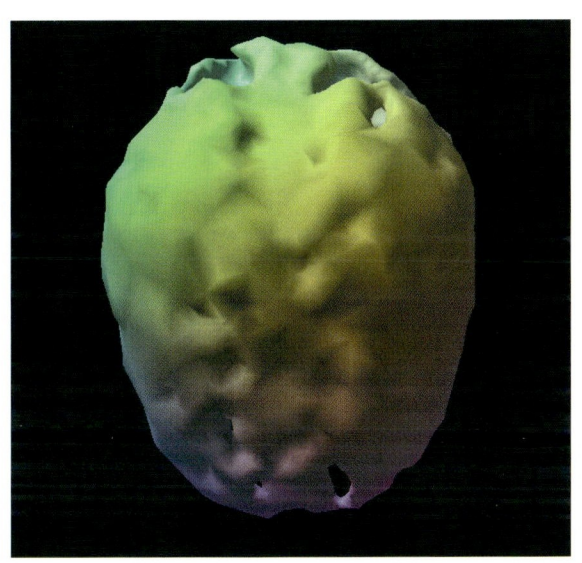

*top down surface view
marked decreased left frontal
prefrontal and occipital lobes*

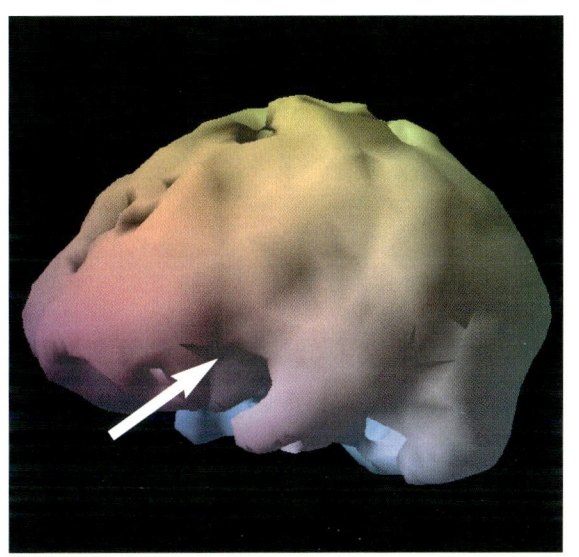

*side surface view
marked decreased left prefrontal
and anterior temporal region*

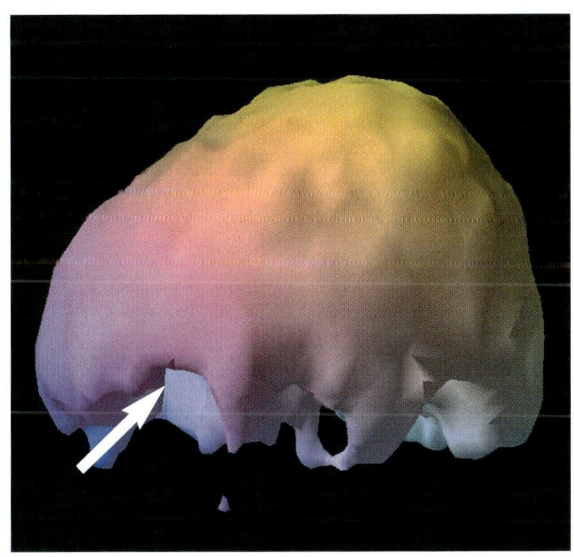

*side surface view
decreased left prefrontal cortex*

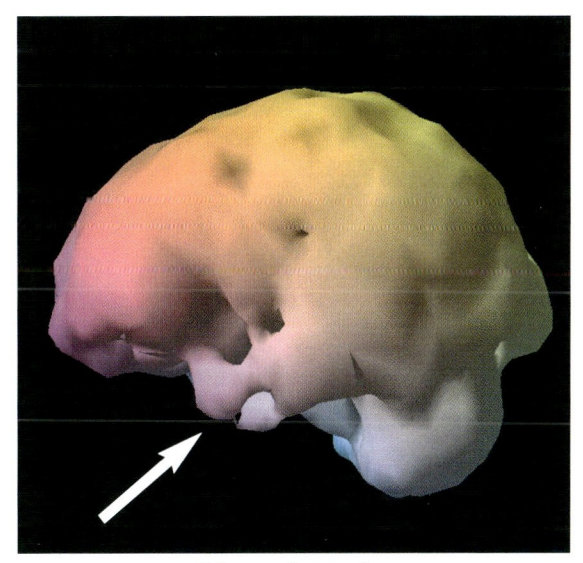

*side surface view
decreased left prefrontal and
temporal lobe activity*

12:7

IMAGES OF HUMAN BEHAVIOR

7. Ring of Fire ADD - many of the children and teenagers who present with symptoms of ADD have the "ring of fire" pattern on SPECT. They often do not respond to psychostimulant medication and in many cases are made worse by them. They tend to improve with either anticonvulsant medications, like Depakote or Neurontin, or the new, novel antipsychotic medications such as Risperdal or Zyprexa. The symptoms of this pattern tend to be severe oppositional behavior, distractibility, irritability and temper problems and mood swings. We think it may represent an early bipolar pattern.

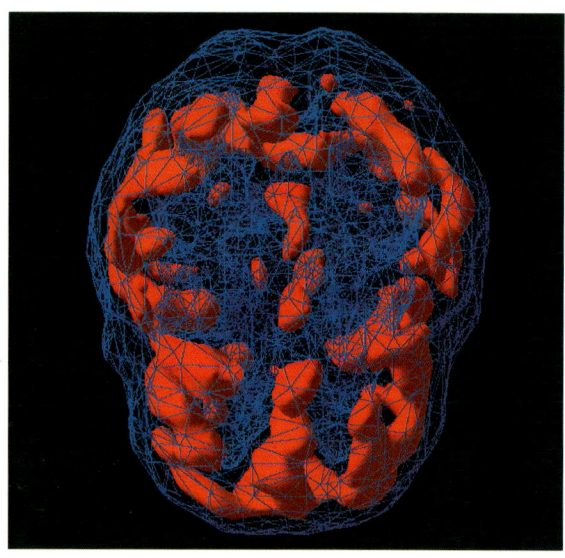

top down active view
increased activity in the anterior cingulate, lateral parietal, frontal and temporal lobes

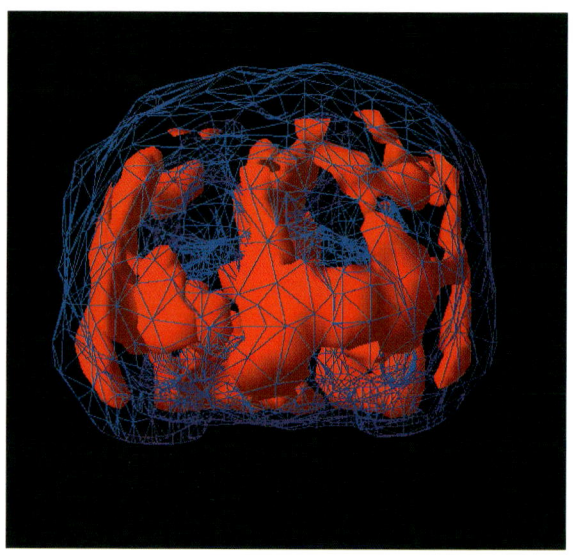

active front on view
increased activity in the anterior cingulate, lateral parietal, frontal and temporal lobes

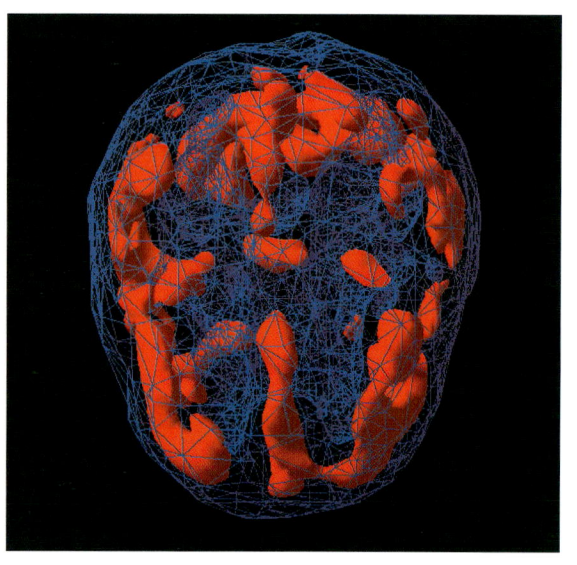

top down active view
increased activity in the anterior cingulate, lateral parietal, frontal and temporal lobes

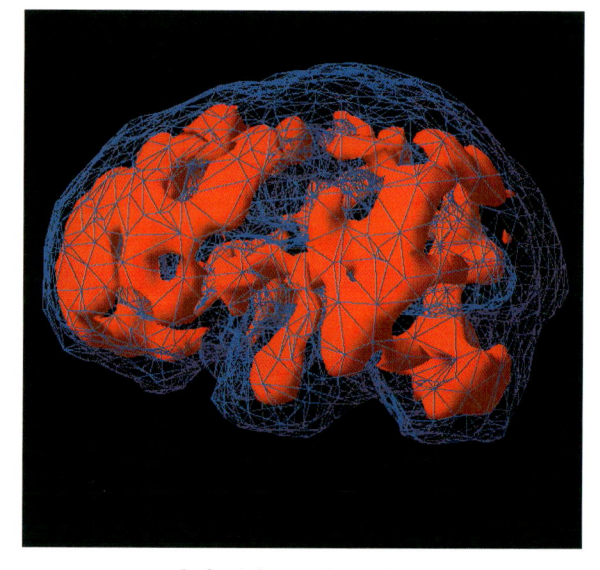

left side active view
increased activity in the anterior cingulate, lateral parietal, frontal and temporal lobes

Section 13

Images of Obsessive Compulsive Spectrum Disorders

There are a number of SPECT studies that report hyperfrontality (increased right and left anterior prefrontal cortex activity and increased anterior cingulate gyrus activity) and increased basal ganglia activity in obsessive compulsive disorder. Of interest, hyperactivity in the anterior cingulate gyrus has also been noticed in oppositional defiant disorder and violence. The anterior cingulate gyrus, which is heavily innervated by serotonergic fibers, has been postulated as being involved with shifting attention and cognitive flexibility, deficient in all of these disorders. Treatment with serotonergic antidepressants such as fluoxetine and clomipramine decrease the hyperactivity in these areas.

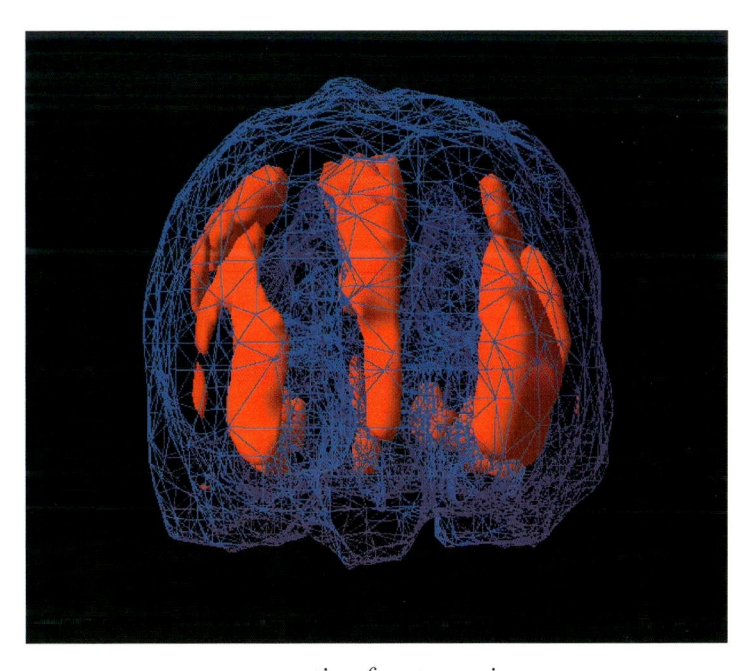

active front-on view
heavy increased anterior cingulate activity and right and left anterior lateral prefrontal cortex activity (together termed hyperfrontality).

OCD

On the outside, Gail was normal. She went to work every day, she was married to her high school sweetheart, and she had two small children. On the inside, Gail felt like a mess. Her husband was ready to leave her and her children were often withdrawn and upset. Gail was distant from her family and locked into the private hell of obsessive compulsive disorder. She cleaned her house for hours every night after work. She screamed at her husband and children when anything was out of place. She would become especially hysterical if she saw a piece of hair on the floor, and she was often at the sink washing her hands. She also made her husband and children wash their hands more than ten times a day. She stopped making love to her husband because she couldn't stand the feeling of being messy.

On the verge of divorce, Gail and her husband came to see me. At first, her husband was very skeptical about the biological nature of her illness. Gail's brain SPECT study showed marked increased activity in the anterior cingulate system, demonstrating that she really did have trouble shifting her attention.

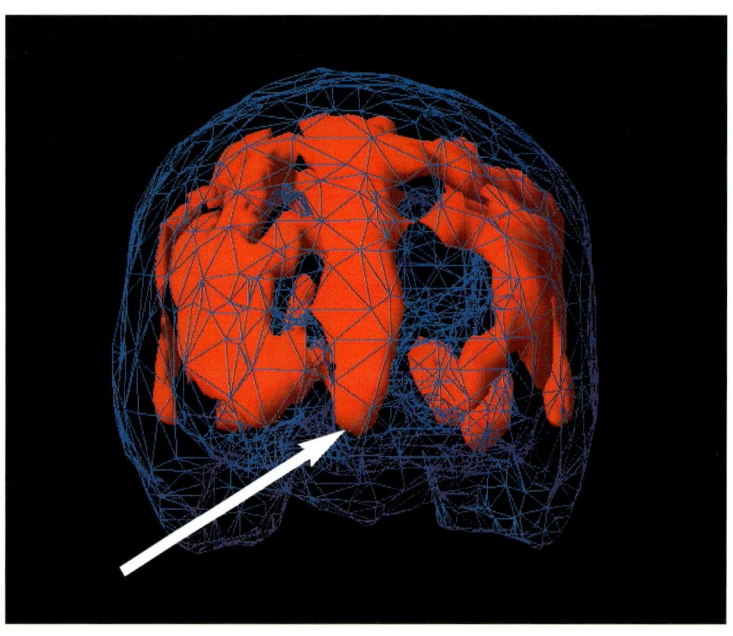

front-on active view
heavy increased anterior cingulate activity

With this information, I placed Gail on Zoloft. Within six weeks, she had significantly relaxed, her ritualistic behavior had diminished and she stopped making her kids wash their hands every time they turned around. Her husband couldn't believe the change. Gail was more like the woman he married.

IMAGES OF HUMAN BEHAVIOR

ODD - Oppositional Defiant Disorder

13-year-old boy with severe oppositional defiant disorder

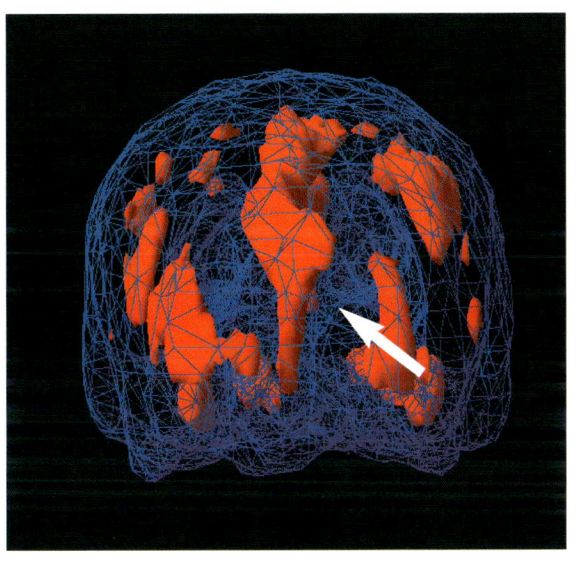

front-on active view

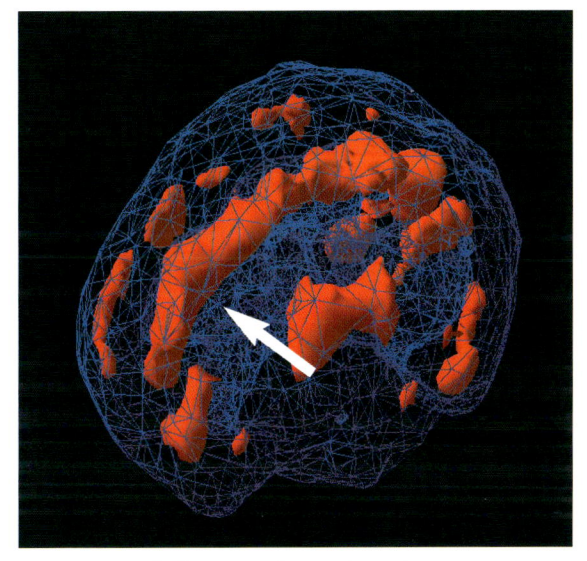

left top-side active view

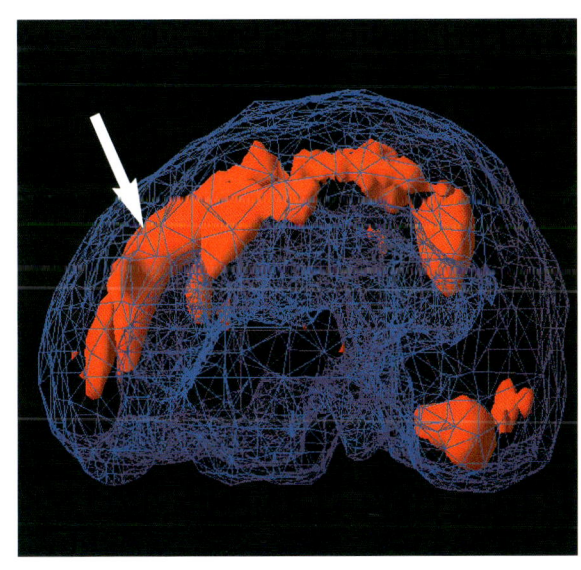

left side active view

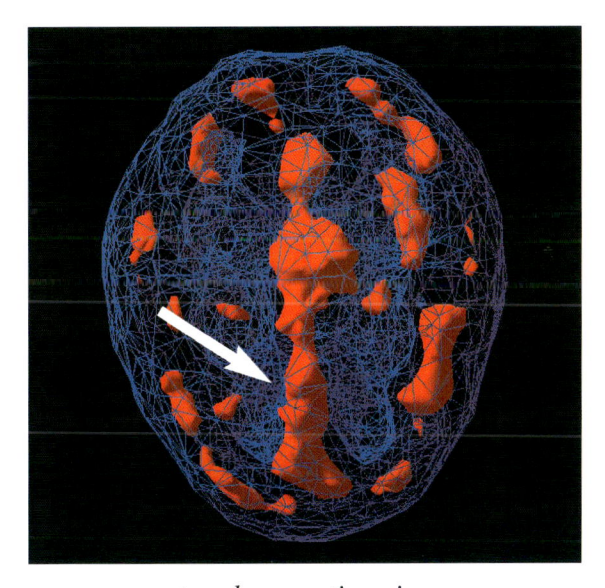

top down active view

Road Rage

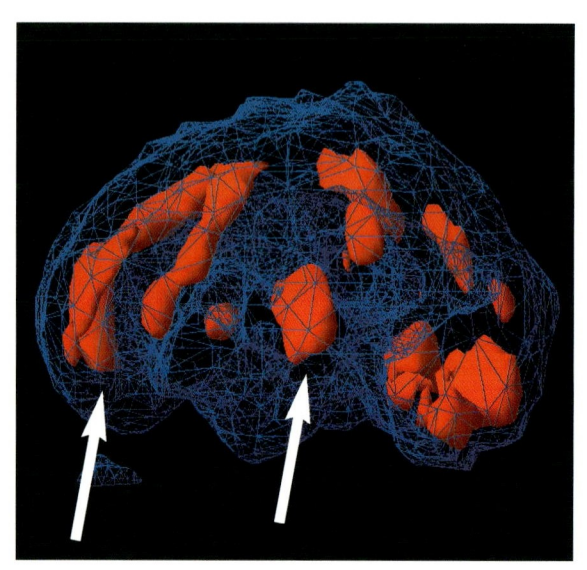

side active view
increased anterior cingulate
and left temporal lobe activity

28-year-old female who has become aggressive while driving on many occassions.

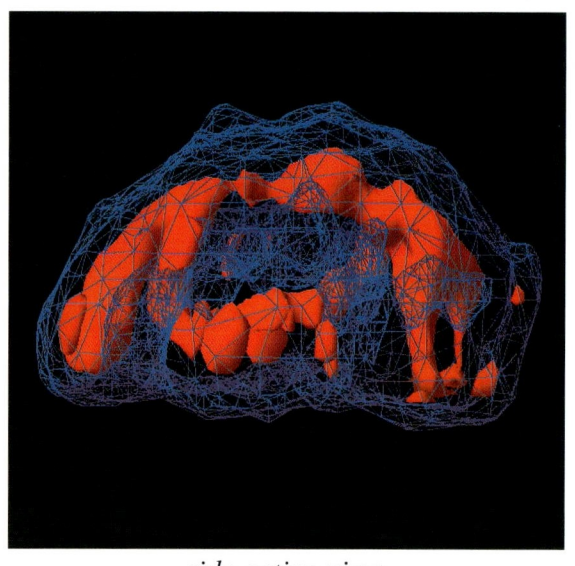

side active view
marked increased anterior cingulate and
left lateral temporal lobe activity

37-year-old male attorney who, on several occasions, chased other drivers who had cut him off and on two occasions got out of the car and bashed their windows in with a baseball bat he kept in the car. After the second incident, he came to see me. He said, "If I don't get help for this I'm sure I'll end up in jail." His cingulate gyrus was markedly overactive, causing him to get locked into the negative thoughts and subsequently be less able to control his frustration. His SPECT scan shows: marked increased activity in the anterior cingulate gyrus and left temporal lobe (arrows), which correlates with irritability and overfocus issues.

Pathological Gambling

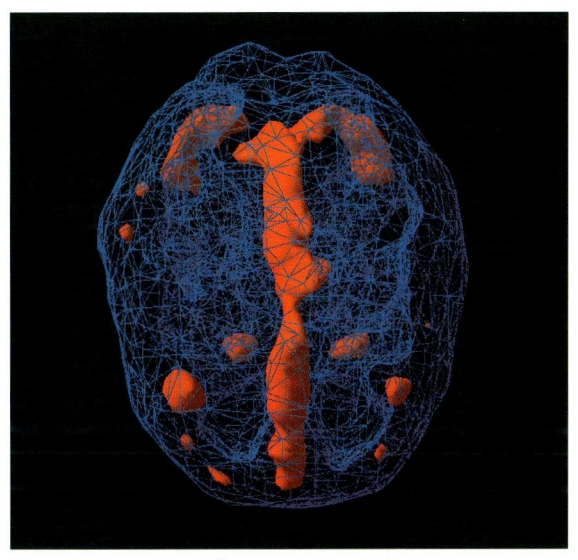

top down active view

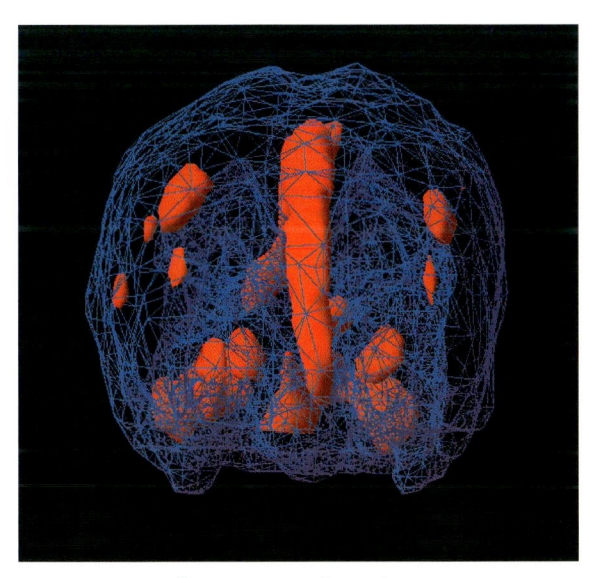

front on active view 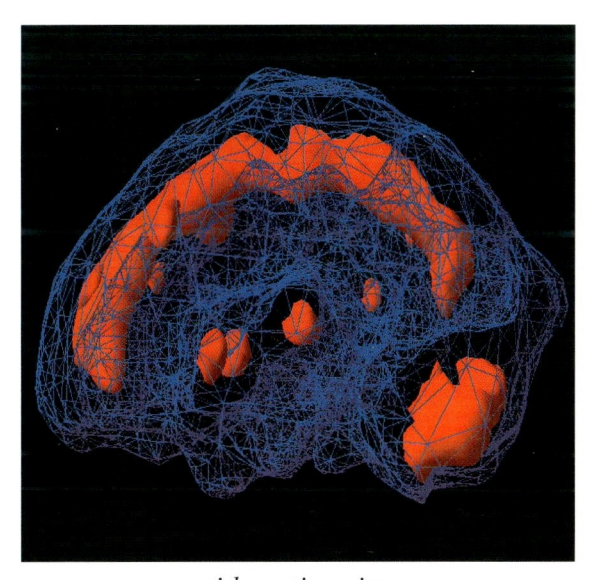 *side active view*

marked increased anterior cingulate activity

Adam came to our office when his wife left him. His gambling had gotten out of control. In the past few years he began neglecting his business spending more of his time at the racetrack and driving back and forth to the casinos in Reno and Lake Tahoe. "I feel compelled to gamble. I know it is ruining my life, but it seems I have to place a bet or the tension just builds and builds. It is all I think about!" Adam's SPECT study showed heavy increased anterior cingulate activity. Explaining the anterior cingulate system to Adam was helpful. He could identify many people in his family who had problems shifting attention. "You should see our family gatherings," he told me, "someone is always mad at someone else. People in my family can hold grudges for years and years." In addition to going to Gamblers Anonymous and being seen in psychotherapy I prescribed a small dose of Prozac for him to help him shift away from the obsessive thoughts about gambling. Eventually, he was able to reconnect with his wife and rebuild his business.

Chronic Pain

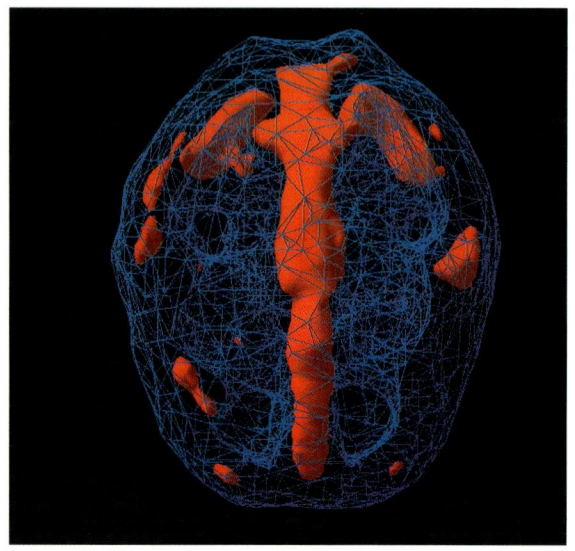

top down active view

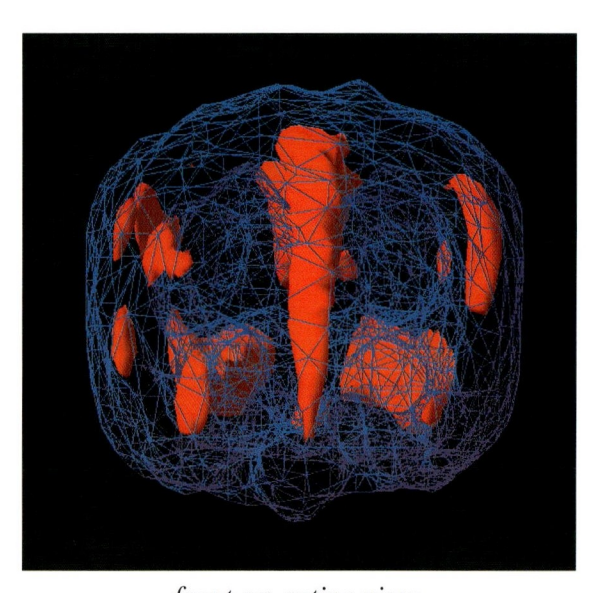

front on active view

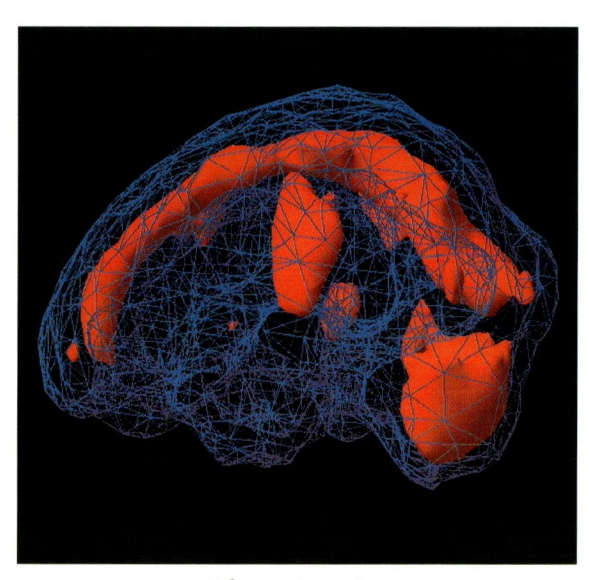

side active view

marked increased anterior cingulate activity

Stewart, a 40-year-old roofer, hurt his back ten years ago when he fell off a roof. He underwent six back operations but remained in constant pain. He was essentially bedridden and about to lose his family because all he could think about was the pain. The threat of losing his family catalyzed him to get a psychiatric evaluation. His SPECT revealed marked overactivity in the anterior cingulate system. He was placed on Anafranil 200 mg a day. After 5 weeks, he reported that his back still hurt, but he was much less focused on the pain. He was able to get out of bed and start back to school. Other researchers have also reported several cases of intractable pain that were also responsive to treatment with anti-obsessive medications.

Section 14

Images of Violence

SPECT can be helpful in understanding and treating aggressive behavior. I have found a consistent triad of SPECT findings common in children, teenagers and adults who exhibit aggressive behavior. These findings include:

- abnormalities (either increased or decreased activity) in the left temporal lobe, often the seat of aggressive thoughts
- increased activity in the anterior cingulate gyrus, which often causes problems with repetitive thoughts and shifting attention (a person may get stuck on the aggressive thoughts that are present) and
- decreased activity in the prefrontal cortex, leading to poor internal supervision.

When these three findings are present it is often helpful to intervene with anticonvulsant medication to stabilize temporal lobe abnormalities and decrease violent thoughts, a serotonergic agent to help decrease anterior cingulate activity and improve cognitive flexibility, and sometimes a psychostimulant to activate prefrontal cortex activity and enhance impulse control.

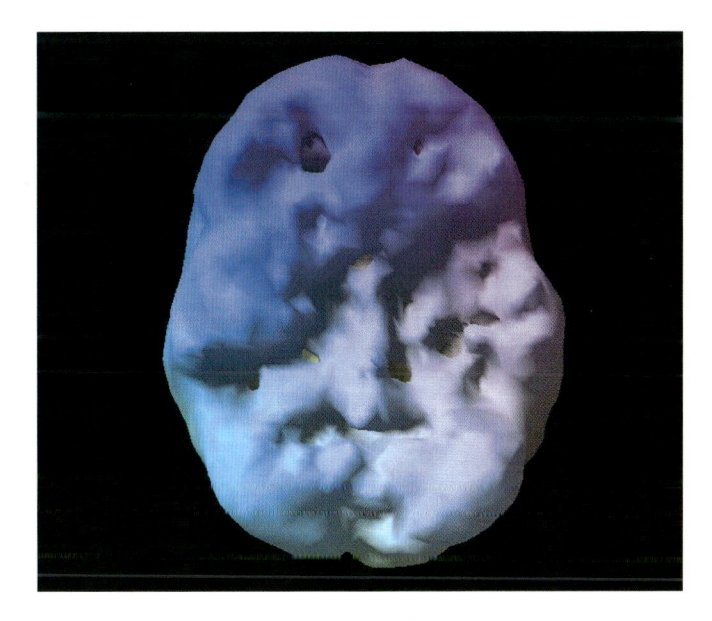

underside surface view
arachnoid cyst occupying the space of the left temporal lobe in a violent 9 year old boy

John

John, a right-handed 79-year-old contractor, had a longstanding history of alcohol abuse and violent behavior. He had frequently physically abused his wife over 40 years of marriage and had been abusive to the children when they were living at home. Almost all of the abuse occurred when he was intoxicated. At age 79, John underwent open-heart surgery. After the surgery he had a psychotic episode, lasting 10 days. His doctor ordered a SPECT study as part of his evaluation. The study showed marked decreased activity in the left outside frontal-temporal region, a finding most likely due to a past head injury. When the doctor asked John if he had ever had any significant head injuries, John told him about a time when he was 20-years-old. While driving an old milk truck, that was missing it's side rear mirror, he put his head out of the window to look behind him. His head struck a pole, knocking him unconscious for several hours. After the head injury he had more problems with his temper and memory. There was a family history of alcohol abuse in 4 of his 5 brothers. None of his brothers had problems with aggressive behavior.

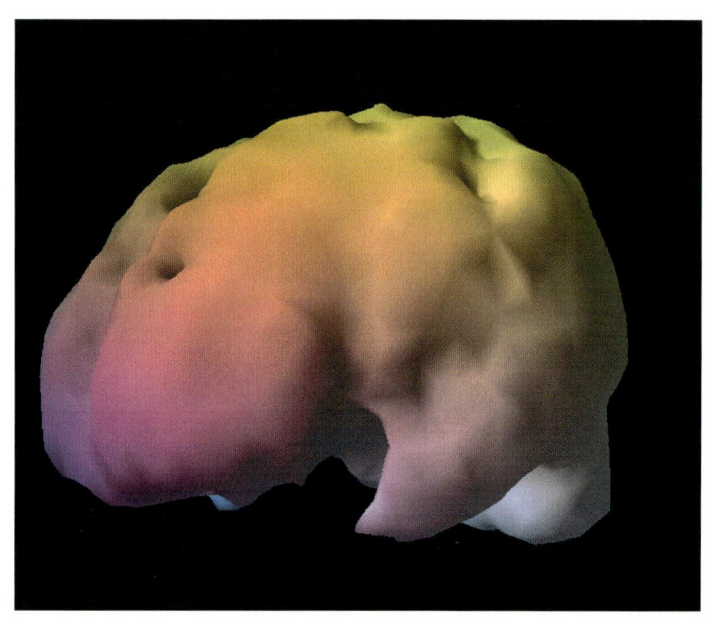

left lateral surface view
note marked area of decreased activity in the left frontal and temporal region

Given the location of the brain abnormalities (left frontal-temporal dysfunction) he was more likely to exhibit violent behavior. The alcohol abuse, which did not elicit violent behavior in his brothers, did in him. Knowing this information earlier might well have been useful in obtaining help for his problems.

Bradley

Bradley was diagnosed with attention deficit/hyperactivity disorder (ADHD) and left temporal lobe dysfunction (diagnosed by EEG) at the age of 14. Before then (from grades 1-8) he had been expelled from 11 schools for fighting, frequently cut school and had already started drinking alcohol and using marijuana. He had a positive response to Ritalin. He improved three grade levels of reading within the next year, attended school regularly and had no aggressive outbursts. However, Bradley had a negative emotional response to taking medication. Two years after starting his medication he decided to stop it on his own without telling anyone. His anger escalated. One night his uncle came to his home and asked Bradley to help him "rob some bitches." Bradley went with his uncle who forced a woman into her car, made her go to her ATM and withdraw money. The uncle and Bradley then raped the woman twice. He was apprehended two weeks later and charged with kidnapping, robbery and rape.

As the psychiatric forensic consultant I ordered a series of brain SPECT studies: the rest study showed mild decreased activity in the left prefrontal cortex and the left temporal lobe. While performing a concentration task there was marked suppression of the prefrontal cortex, a finding common in attention deficit hyperactivity disorder and both temporal lobes. A third scan was done one hour after taking 15 mg. of methylphenidate. This scan showed marked activation in the prefrontal cortex and both temporal lobes, although there was still some mild deactivation in the left temporal lobe. After understanding the history and reviewing the scan data it was apparent that Bradley already had a vulnerable brain that was consistent with long-term behavioral and academic difficulties. His substance use may have further suppressed an already underactive prefrontal cortex and temporal lobe diminishing executive abilities and unleashing aggressive tendencies. It is possible that with an explanation of the underlying metabolic problems and brief psychotherapy on the emotional issues surrounding the need to take medication this serious problem might have been averted.

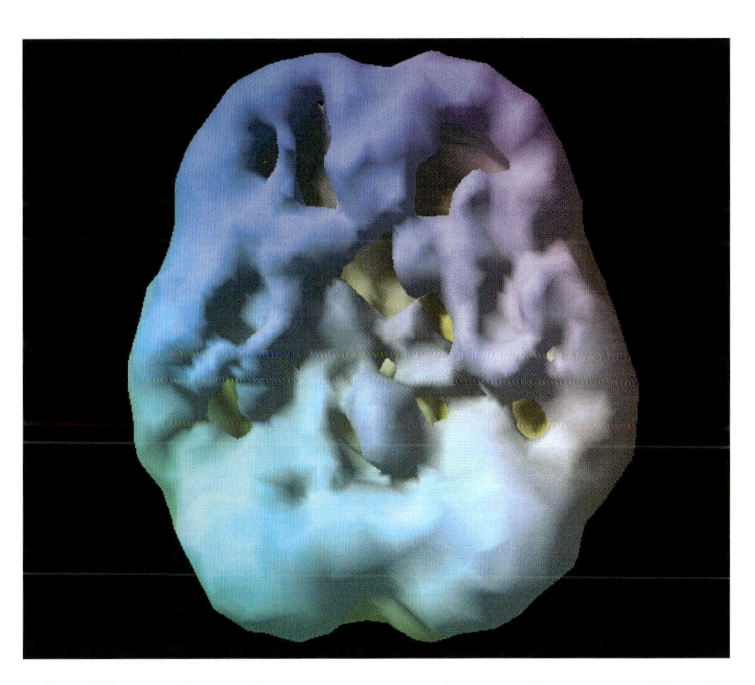

underside surface view, concentration study, no medication
marked decreased prefrontal and temporal lobe activity

Rusty

Twenty-eight-year-old Rusty had a severe methamphetamine problem. He was unable to keep steady work, he was involved in a physically abusive relationship with his girlfriend (arrested four times for assault and battery), he was mean to his parents even though they tried to help him. He failed five drug treatment programs. Since Rusty's mom scheduled his SPECT study he was unaware of it until the morning of the scan. He showed up loaded with a gram of methamphetamine from the night before. Rusty told me about his drug abuse. I decided to scan Rusty that morning with the effects of the methamphetamine still in his system and then a week later off all drugs. When Rusty was under the influence of high dose methamphetamine his brain looked suppressed in activity. A week later, however, off all drugs, he had a terribly hot (overactive) left temporal lobe, probably causing his problems with violent behavior. Rusty was likely self-medicating an underlying temporal lobe problem with high dose methamphetamine. Given this finding, I put Rusty on Tegretol (an anti-seizure medication, which stabilizes activity in the temporal lobes). Within 2 weeks Rusty felt better than he had in years. He was calmer, his temper was under control and for the first time in his life he was able to remain gainfully employed. An additional benefit of the scan was that I showed Rusty the serious damage he was doing to his brain by abusing the methamphetamines. Even though the drugs helped his temporal lobe problem, they were clearly toxic to his brain.

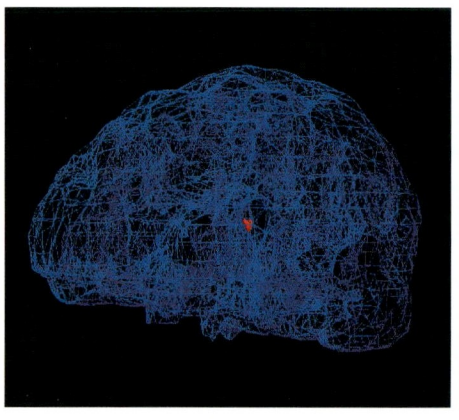

active side view
on high dose metamphetamine

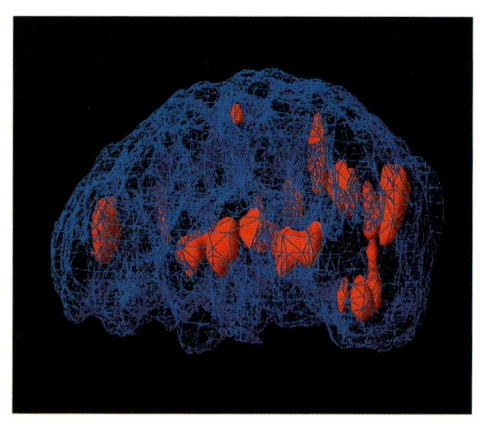

active side view
off metamphetamine

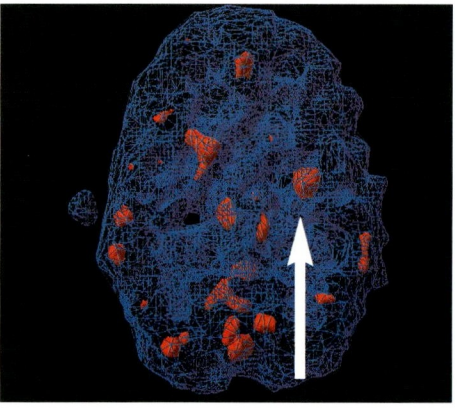

underside active view
notice hot area deep left temporal lobe

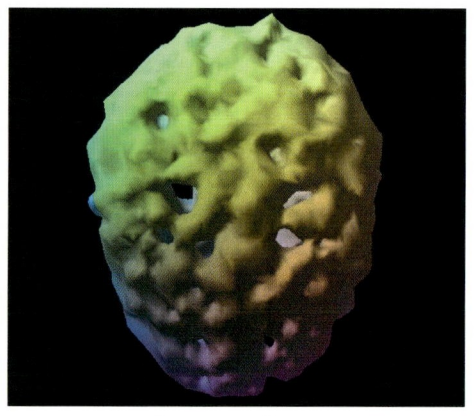

top-down surface view
notice multiple holes across cortex

Jose

Jose, a 16-year-old gang member, was arrested after he and another gang member beat another teenager nearly to death. They were charged with attempted murder. Their gang claimed the color red. One evening, when they were in an intoxicated state (from both alcohol and heavy marijuana usage), they approached a boy who was wearing a red sweater walking his dog across the street. They asked him, "What colors do you bang?" (asking him about his gang affiliation). When the boy said he did not know what they were talking about Jose replied, "Wrong answer," and the two gang boys started to physically attack the boy, hitting and kicking him repeatedly until he was unconscious. The public defender ordered neuropsychological testing on Jose which found frontal lobe dysfunction and evidence of ADHD, depression and learning disabilities. The psychologist suggested a resting and concentration SPECT series for independent verification. The SPECT series was significantly abnormal. Both studies showed marked increased activity in the cingulate gyrus, consistent with problems shifting attention. At rest, his SPECT also showed mildly suppressed prefrontal cortex activity. While doing a concentration task there was also marked suppression of the prefrontal cortex and both temporal lobes, consistent with ADHD, learning disabilities and aggressive tendencies.

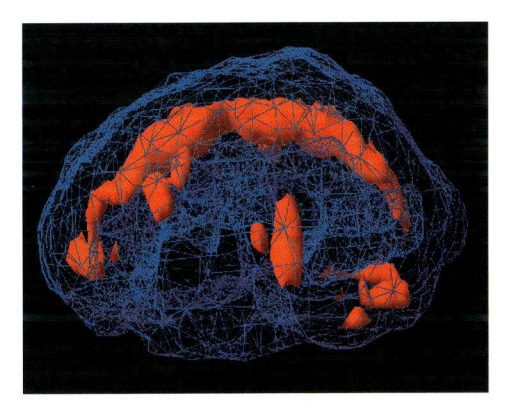

left side active view
marked increased
whole cingulate gyrus

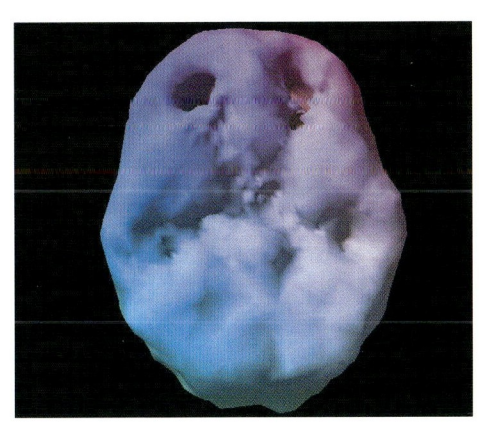

at rest
mild decreased pfc activity

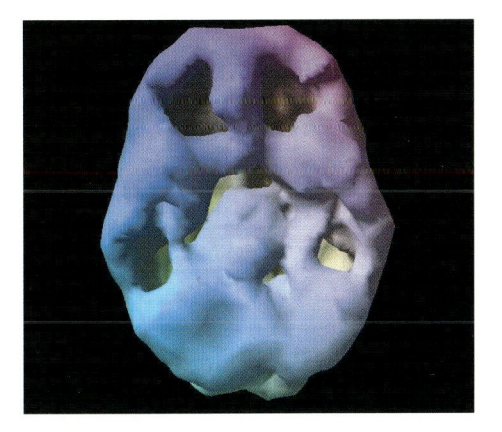

during concentration
marked decreased pfc and temporal lobe activity

Paul

Paul, a 28-year-old gardener, came to my clinic for work-related problems. He had increasingly intense feelings of rage toward his boss. Paul said that his boss was prejudiced against him because he was Hispanic. He frequently thought about killing his boss. He reported that only the thought of his wife and small daughter prevented him from doing physical harm to his boss. He needed to maintain his job in order to support his family. Paul could not get the anger toward his boss out of his head. He reported that since childhood he had many explosive outbursts. He saw himself as someday being on the top of a tower shooting down at people. His anger was diffuse. He described himself as having an extremely short fuse, especially while driving. At the age of 7 he ran full speed into a metal basketball pole and was unconscious for several minutes. Paul had no evidence of a psychotic disorder or a significant depression, although he did complain of short periods of confusion, fear for no reason and episodes of deja vu. His EEG was within normal limits. A brain SPECT study was obtained in order to further evaluate any underlying brain abnormalities that might have been contributing to his difficulties.

Paul's brain SPECT study was significantly abnormal. It revealed normal activity in the prefrontal cortex at rest that worsened when he tried to concentrate (problems with impulsivity). There was also moderate marked increased uptake in the deep aspects of the left temporal lobe (short fuse) and his cingulate gyrus (stuck on thoughts). Because of the clinical picture and information from the brain SPECT study Paul was placed on the anticonvulsant Tegretol at therapeutic levels, along with Prozac several weeks later. After six weeks, he reported that he noted a sense of increased inner control and inner peace. His periods of confusion, deja vu and fearfulness diminished. His anger outbursts decreased and he was able to go to work at a new job.

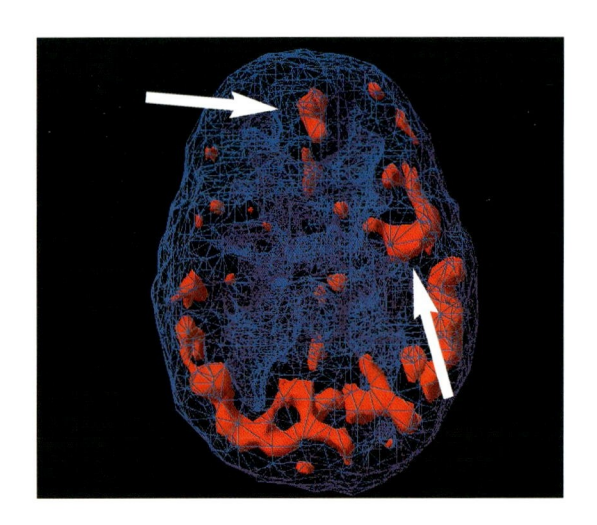

underside active view

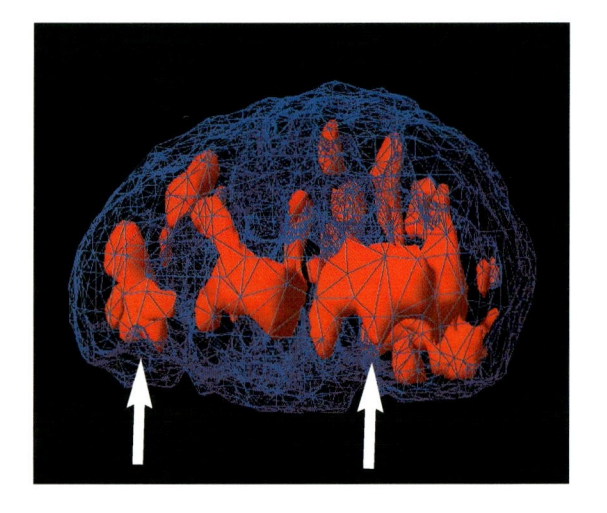

left side active view

note marked increased activity in the left temporal lobe and anterior cingulate (arrows)

Steven

Steven, a 39-year-old radio station engineer, was admitted to the hospital for suicidal thoughts. He was recently separated from his wife of eight years. During their relationship there had been mutual physical spousal abuse for which he had spent some time in jail. Steven also complained of having a very "short fuse." He found himself frequently yelling at other drivers on the road and was easily upset at work. On admission he was tearful, had problems sleeping and poor concentration. He was depressed and experienced suicidal thoughts. He reported short periods of confusion, intense rage with little provocation, and episodic periods where he would see shadows out of the corners of his eyes. His EEG was within normal limits.

Steven's brain SPECT study revealed marked increased uptake in the deeper aspects of the left temporal lobe and marked increased activity in the cingulate gyrus.

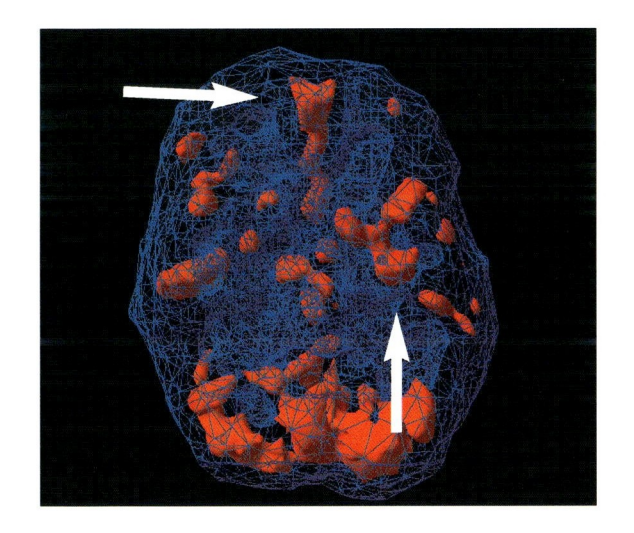

underside active view 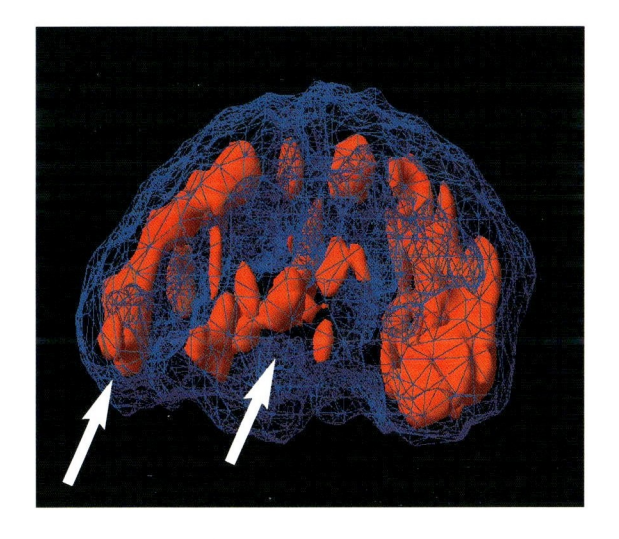   *left side active view*

note marked increased activity in the left temporal lobe and anterior cingulate (arrows)

With the clinical picture and information from the brain SPECT it was decided to start Steven on an anticonvulsant in addition to an antidepressant. He was placed on Tegretol at therapeutic levels along with Prozac. Even though he continued to feel sad about the break up of his marriage, he felt calmer, in better self-control and his suicidal thoughts abated. He did report that he wished he had known about the dysfunction in his temporal lobe years earlier. He felt it might have changed the outcome of his marriage.

Jody

In December 1996 Jody Gordon walked into the McDonald's in Vallejo, California where he had been fired from his job the year before. He carried two guns and a knife. Three teenage girls, employees of McDonald's, were sitting at a table having a snack after a meeting they had been called into work. Jody asked the manager for his job back. When the manager refused, Jody walked over to the girls and started shooting. He killed one of the girls and wounded the other two.

As part of his defense I was asked to perform a brain SPECT study to evaluate his brain function. He had one of the most severe decreases in prefrontal cortex function I had ever seen. I then had him come back for a second scan and gave him 20 milligrams of Adderall to see if I could enhance the severe prefrontal hypoperfusion. To my amazement, the Adderall significantly enhanced the activity in his brain, especially in his prefrontal cortex. I wondered if he would have committed this terrible crime if he had more access to the part of his brain involved in decision making.

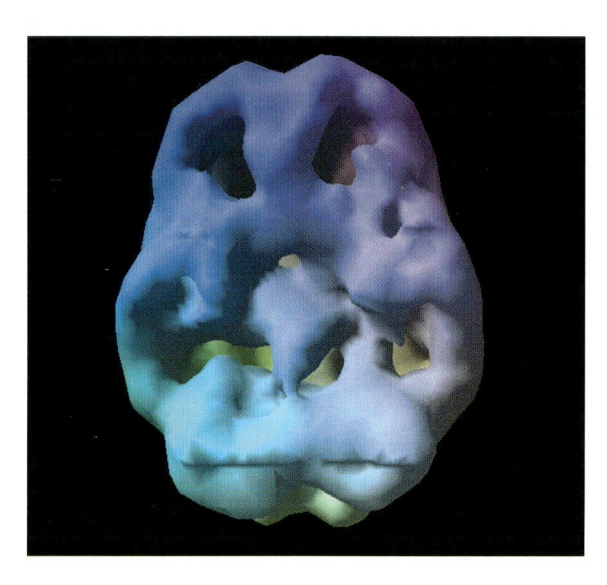

underside surface view, NO MEDS
very poor pfc activity

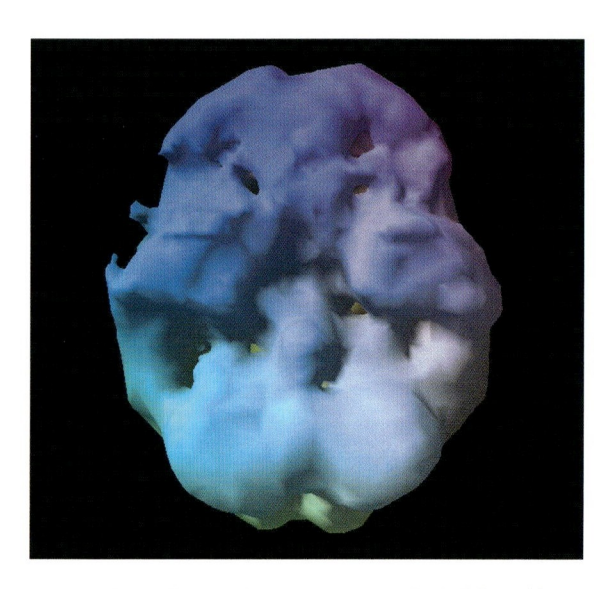

underside surface view, with Adderall
improved pfc, especially on left side

15-year-old male, with a serious head injury,
convicted of raping his girlfriend.

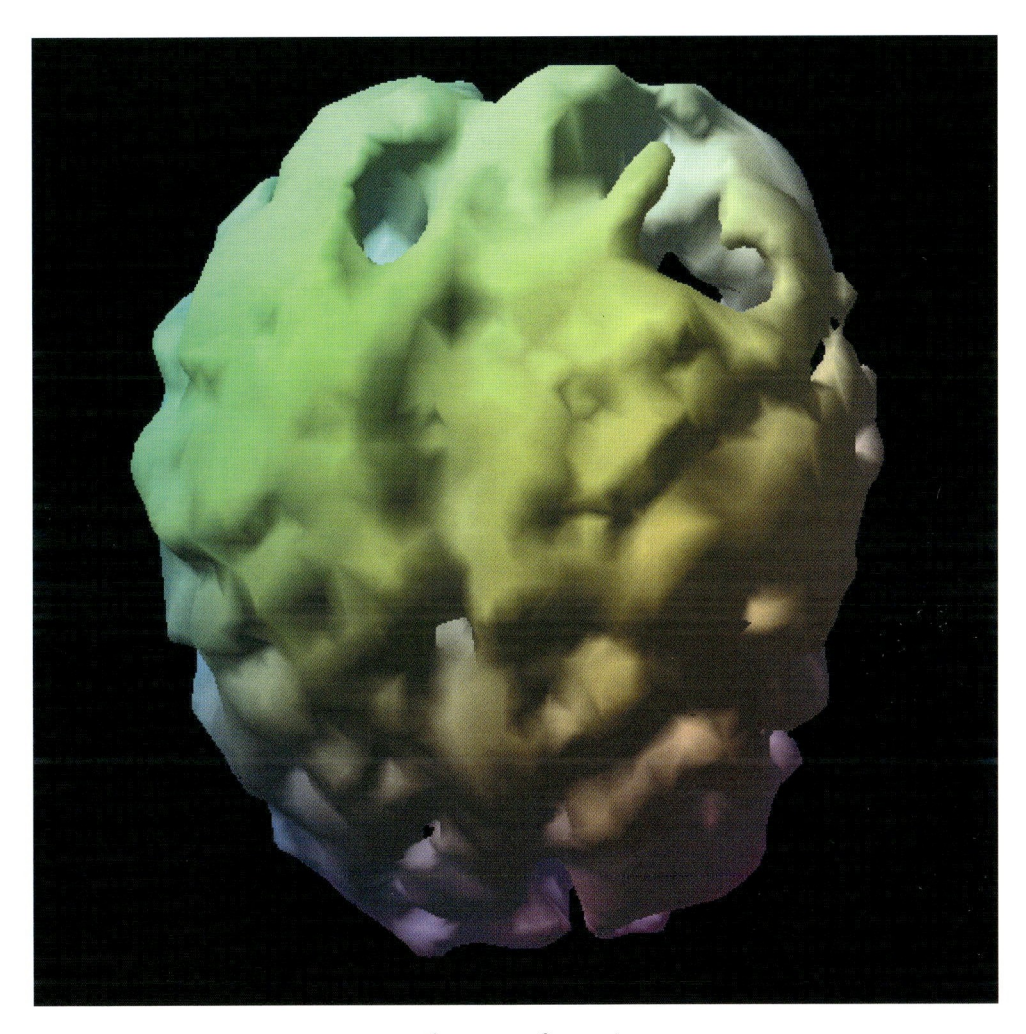

top down surface view
marked damage to the left hemisphere

SECTION 15

Images of Alcohol and Drug Abuse

Brain Pollution and the Real Reason You Shouldn't Use

Studying the effects of drugs and alcohol on the brain has clearly been one of the most informative and fascinating parts of my work. I had a sense growing up that drugs and alcohol weren't helpful to my overall health. I might add, this notion was helped along by getting drunk on a six pack of Michelob and half a bottle of champagne when I was sixteen years old – I was sick for three days. After that, I've been lucky enough to stay away from drugs and alcohol. After doing this work there's no way you could get me to do marijuana, heroin, cocaine, methamphetamine, LSD, PCP, inhalants or any more than a glass or two of wine or beer. These substances damage the patterns in your brain, and without your brain you are not you.

There is really quite a bit of scientific literature on the physiological effects of drugs and alcohol on the brain. SPECT has demonstrated a number of abnormalities in substance abusers in brain areas known to be involved in behavior, such as the frontal and temporal lobes. There are some SPECT similarities and differences between the damage we see caused by the different substances of abuse. I'll discuss the differences in drug abuse patterns below. There tends to be several similarities seen among classes of abused drugs. The most common similarity among drug and alcohol abusers is that the brain has an overall toxic look to it. In general, the SPECT studies look less active, more shriveled, and overall less healthy. A "scalloping effect" is common amongst drug abusing brains. Normal brain patterns show smooth activity across the cortical surface. Scalloping is a wavy, rough sea-like look on the brain's surface. I also see this pattern in patients who have been exposed to toxic fumes or oxygen deprivation. My research assistant says that the drug brains she has seen look like someone poured acid on the brain. Not a pretty site.

SPECT can be helpful in evaluating the effects of drugs and alcohol on the brain. On 3D surface images several substances of abuse appear to show consistent patterns. For example, cocaine and methamphetamine abuse appear as multiple small holes across the cortical surface; heroin abuse appears as marked decreased activity across the whole cortical surface; heavy marijuana abuse shows decreased activity in the temporal lobes bilaterally and heavy alcohol abuse shows marked decreased activity throughout the brain. These findings tend to improve with abstinence, although long-term use has been associated with continued SPECT deficits seen years after abstinence. SPECT can be helpful in several ways in drug and alcohol abuse. First, 3D surface SPECT images of drug and alcohol abusers can be used in drug prevention education. Second, SPECT studies can help break though the denial that often accompanies substance abuse. When one is faced with their own abnormal cerebral perfusion it is hard to remain in denial. Third, SPECT may help evaluate if there is an underlying neuropsychiatric condition that needs treatment.

Marijuana

In our experience, marijuana usage typically causes decreased activity in the posterior temporal lobes bilaterally. The damage can be mild or severe, depending on how long a person used, how much use occurred, what other substances were used (nicotine is a powerful vasoconstrictor) and how vulnerable a particular brain is. For more information see Dr. Amen's article High Resolution Brain SPECT Imaging in Marijuana Smokers with AD/HD, Journal of Psychoactive Drugs, Volume 30, No. 2 April-June 1998. Pgs 1-13.

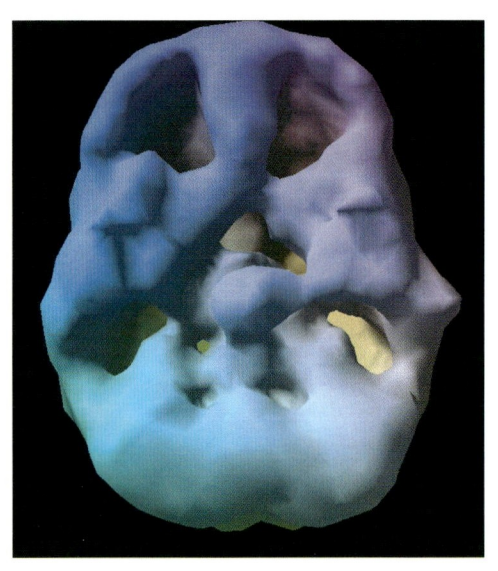

18 y/o–3 year history of 4 x week use
underside surface view
decreased pfc and temporal lobe activity

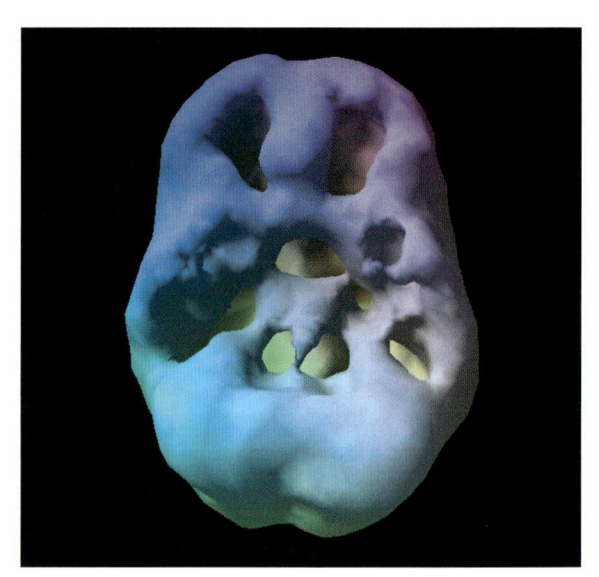

16 y/o–2 year history of daily abuse
underside surface view
decreased pfc and temporal lobe activity

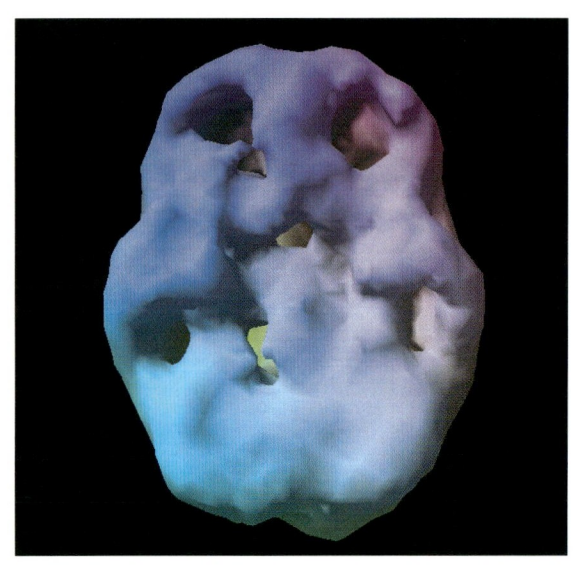

38 y/o–12 years of daily use
underside surface view
decreased pfc and temporal lobe activity

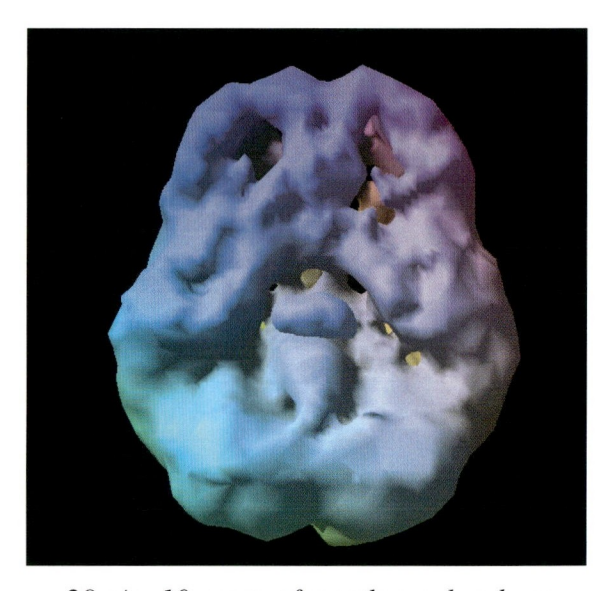

28 y/o–10 years of mostly weekend use
underside surface view
decreased pfc and temporal lobe activity

Off and On Marijuana

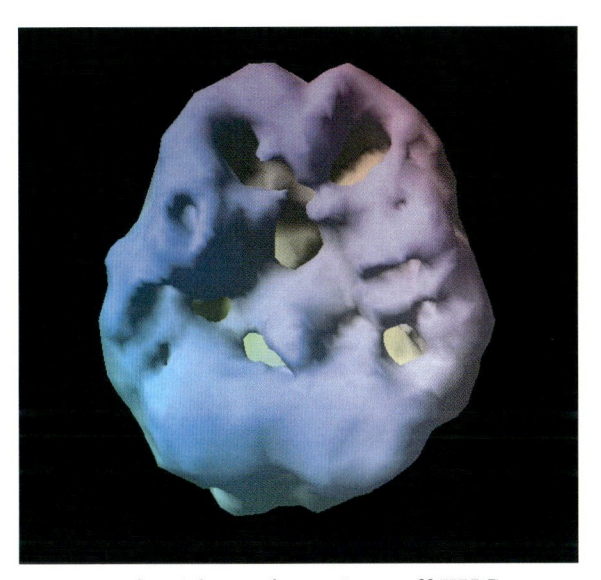

underside surface view, off THC
decreased pfc and temporal lobe activity

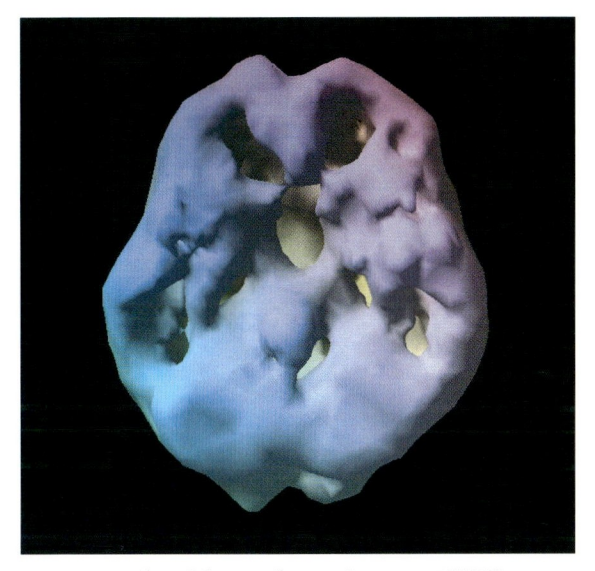

underside surface view, on THC
severe overall decreased activity

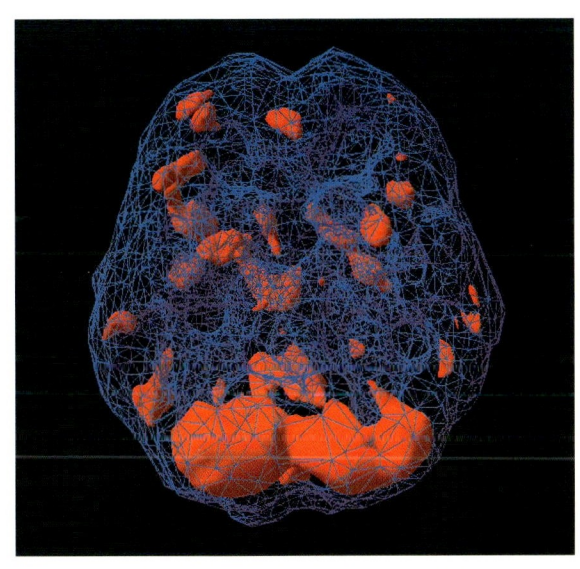

underside active view, off THC
increased deep left temporal lobe activity

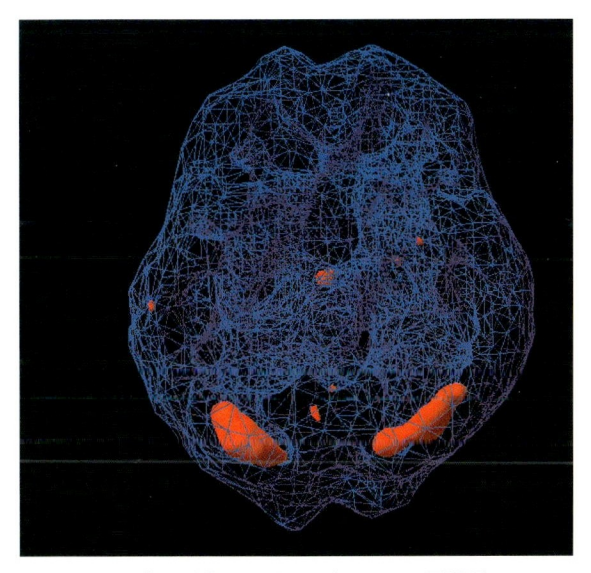

underside active view, on THC
overall calming of activity

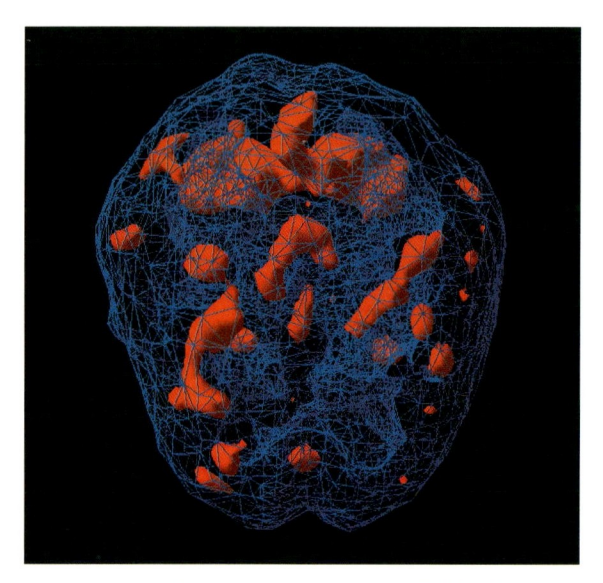

top-down active view, off THC
patchy increased uptake

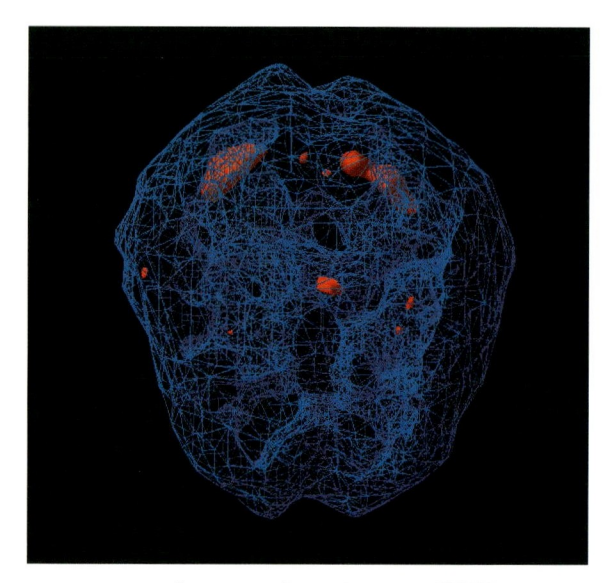

top-down active view, on THC
overall calming of activity

This 57-year-old physician had abused marijuana for 30 years. We performed this SPECT series because he had been unable to stop using without feeling very angry, irritable, agitated and anxious.

The first study (those images in the right column) was performed after he came to the clinic intoxicated from 3 straight days of heavy usage. The second study (those images in the left column) was performed after he abstained from marijuana usage for 1 month.

Notice the study without marijuana shows decreased temporal lobe activity (likely from the chronic marijuana usage), but also patchy increased uptake, especially increased activity in the deep left temporal lobe (often associated with anger, irritability and anxiety). The study with heavy marijuana usage shows marked overall decreased activity, especially in the prefrontal cortex and temporal lobes (associated with attention, memory and motivational problems) but also there is a decrease in the overactive areas noted in the "off marijuana" study.

This scan series argues for the possibility of "self-medication," but unfortunately this medication has the side effect of causing the potential for long-term damage to his brain.

Heroin & Methadone

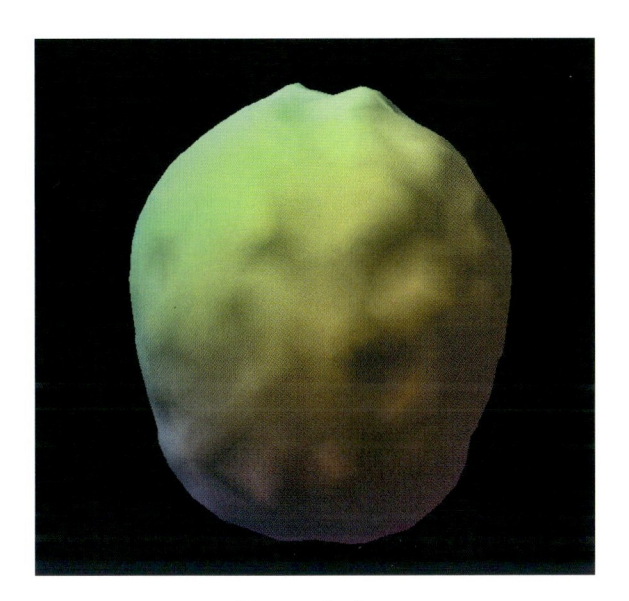

Normal view
top down surface view
full, symmetrical activity

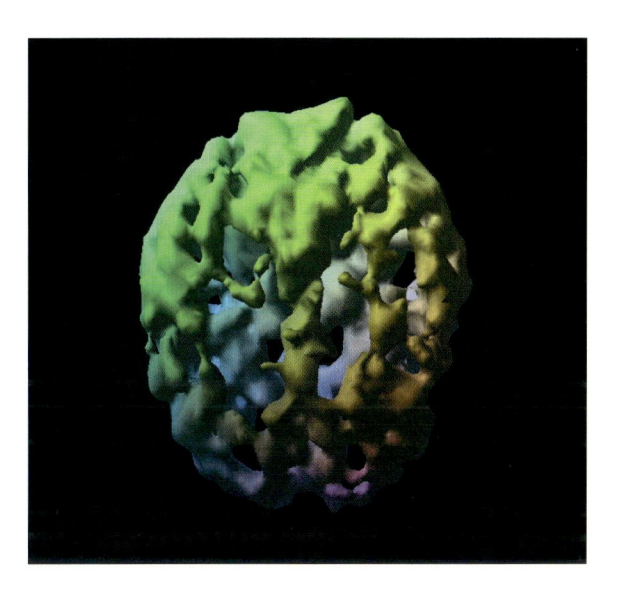

39 y/o–25 yr hx of frequent heroin use
top down surface view
marked overall decreased activity

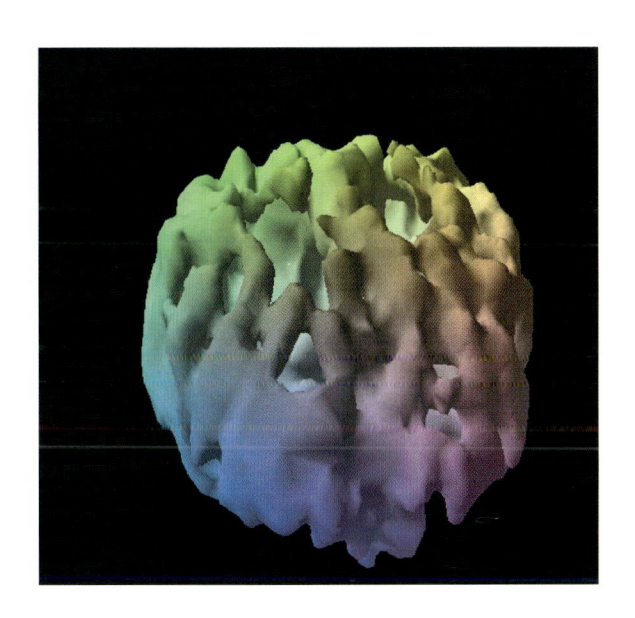

39 y/o–25 yrs of frequent heroin use
front on surface view
marked overall decreased activity

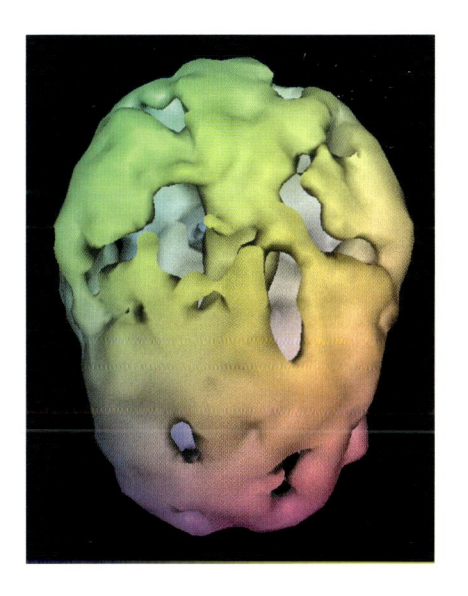

40 y/o–7 yrs on methadone
heroin 10 yrs prior
top down surface view
marked decreased overall activity

Cocaine & Methamphetamine

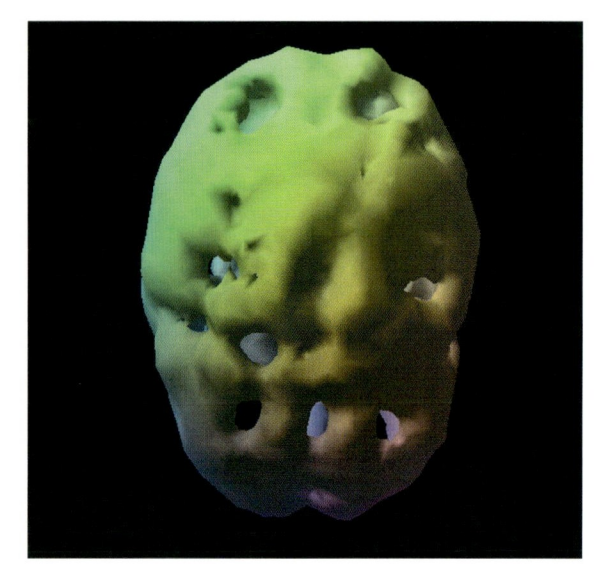

52 y/o–28 yr hx frequent meth use
top down surface view
multiple holes across cortical surface

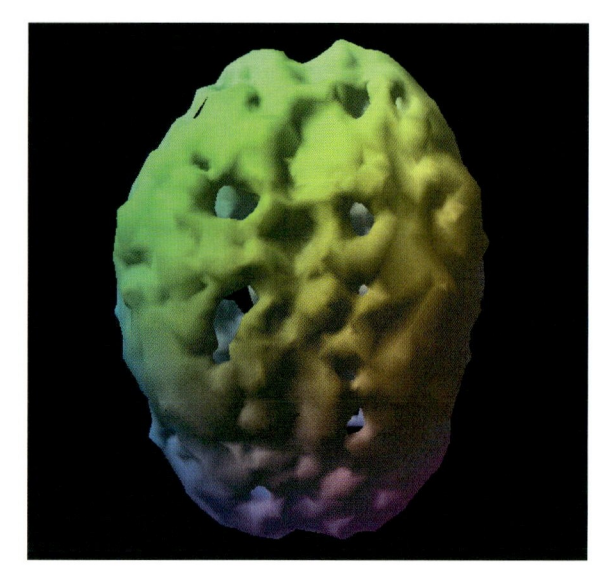

24 y/o–2 yr hx of frequent cocaine use
top down surface view
multiple holes across cortical surface

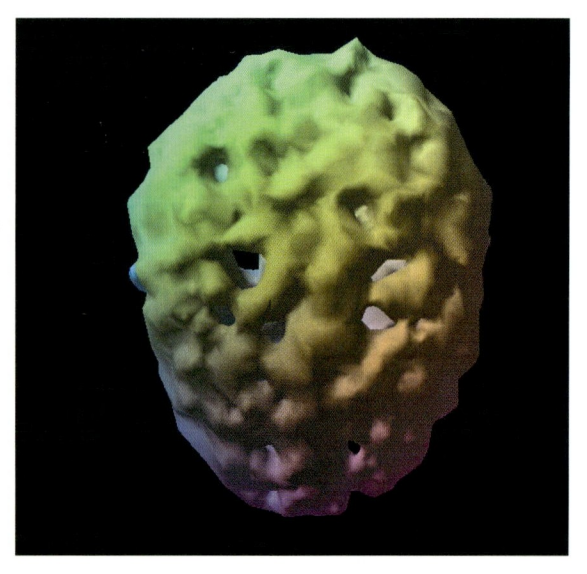

28 y/o–8 yrs heavy meth use
top down surface view
marked overall decreased activity

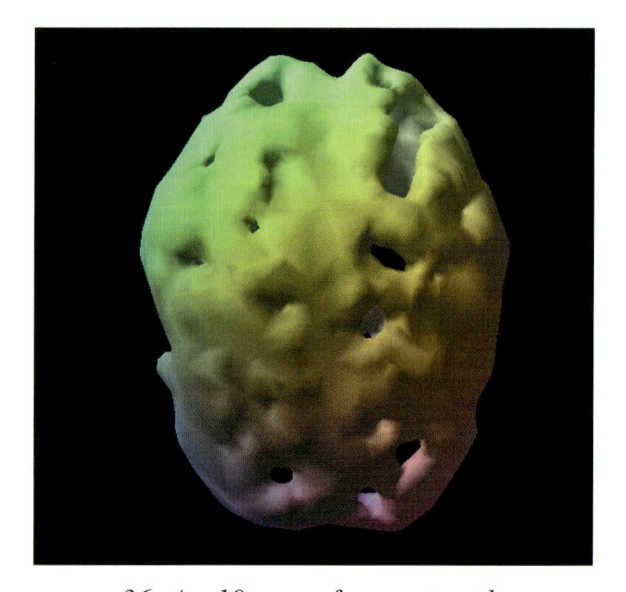

36 y/o–10 years frequent meth
top down surface view
multiple holes across cortical surface

Alcohol
38 y/o–17 years of heavy weekend use

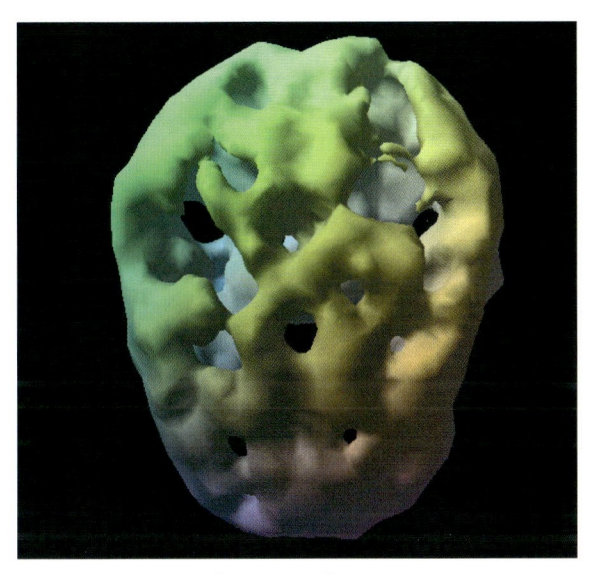

top down surface view

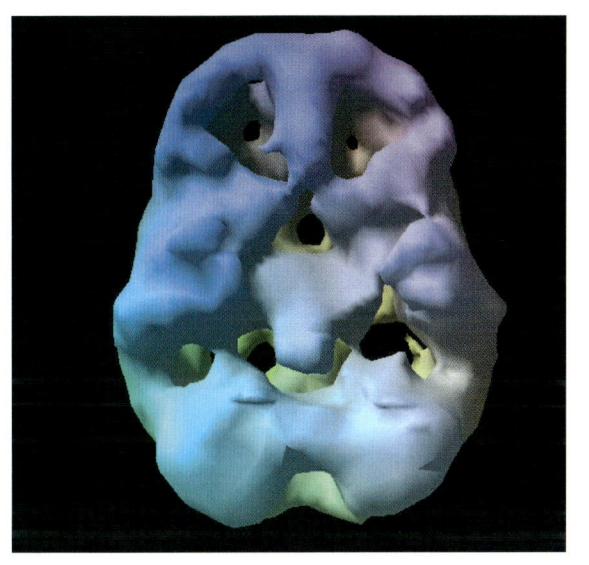

underside surface view

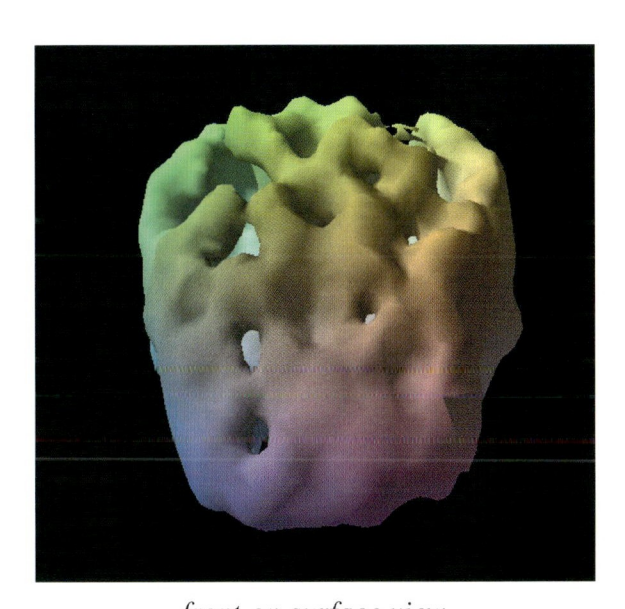

front on surface view

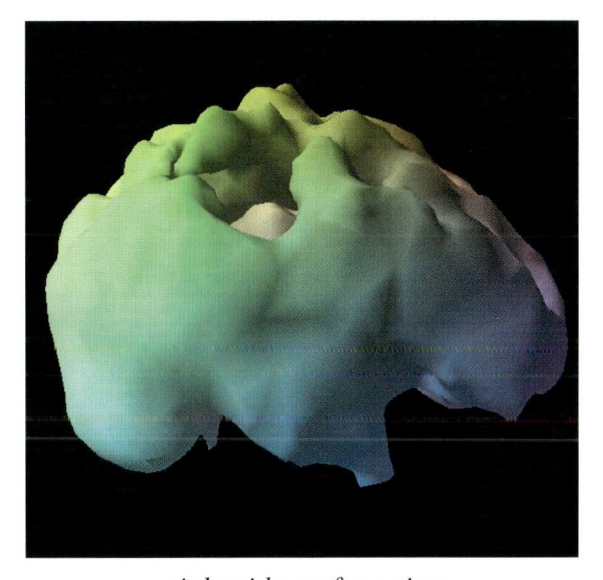

right side surface view

marked overall decreased activity

Alcohol

48 y/o–22 years of daily use with history of past head injury

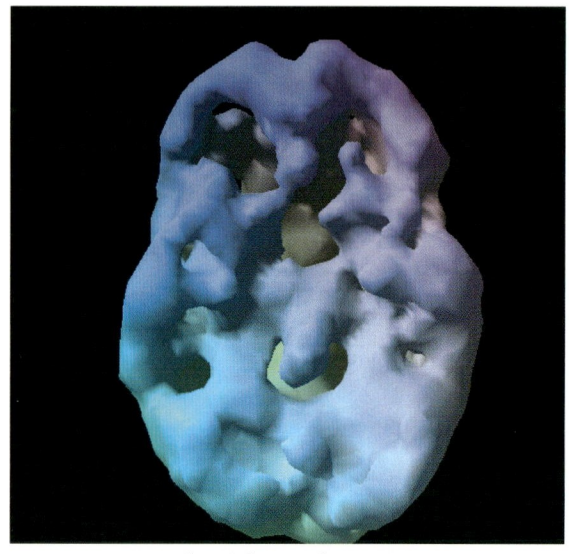

underside surface view 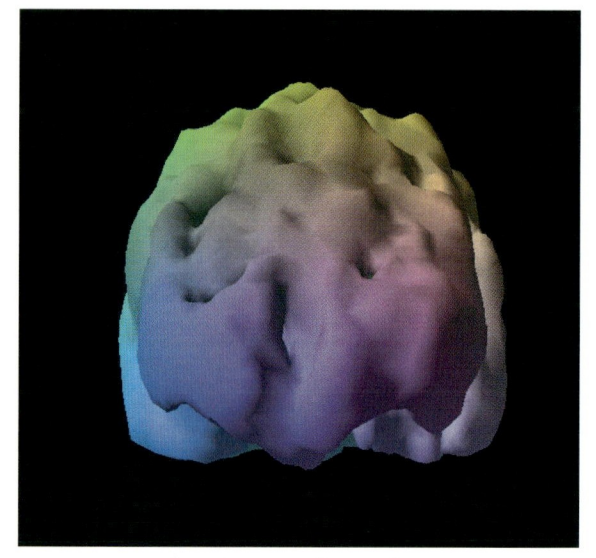   *front on surface view*

marked scalloping overall decreased activity

44 y/o–18 years of daily use

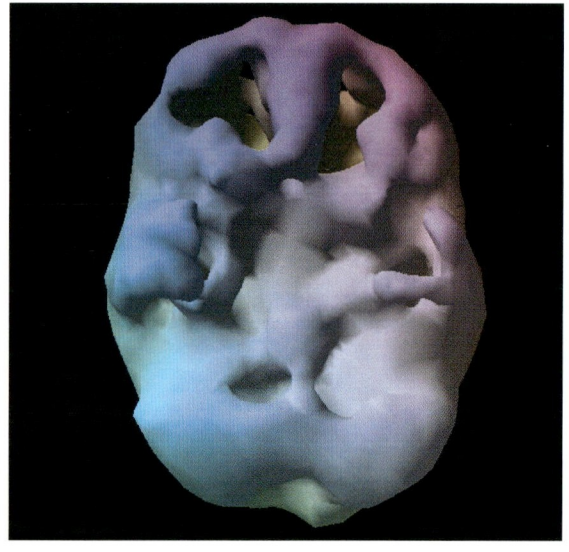

underside surface view
marked overall decreased activity

45 y/o–25-year history of daily abuse

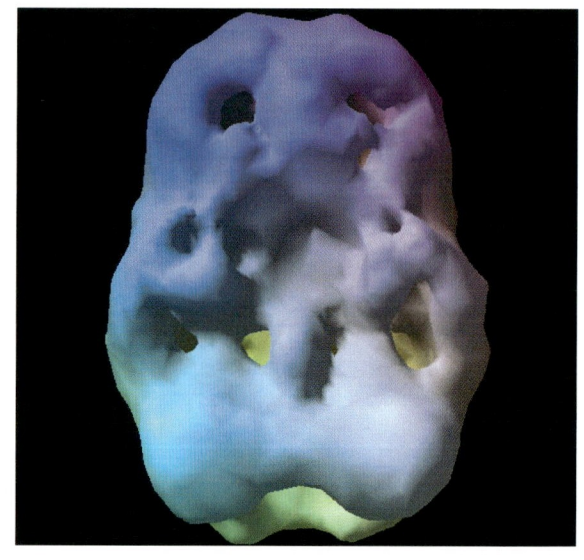

underside surface view
marked overall decreased activity

Images of Alcohol and Drug Abuse

15:8

Hope for Healing
Alcohol, Cocaine & Meth
On and Off Drugs

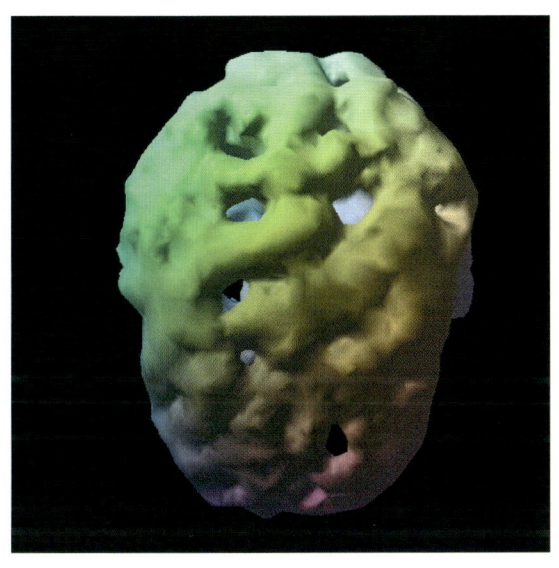

top-down surface view
during substance abuse

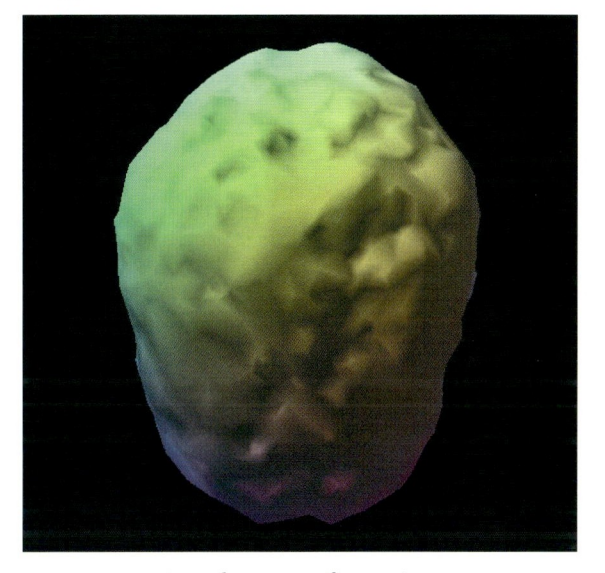

top-down surface view
a year drug and alcohol free

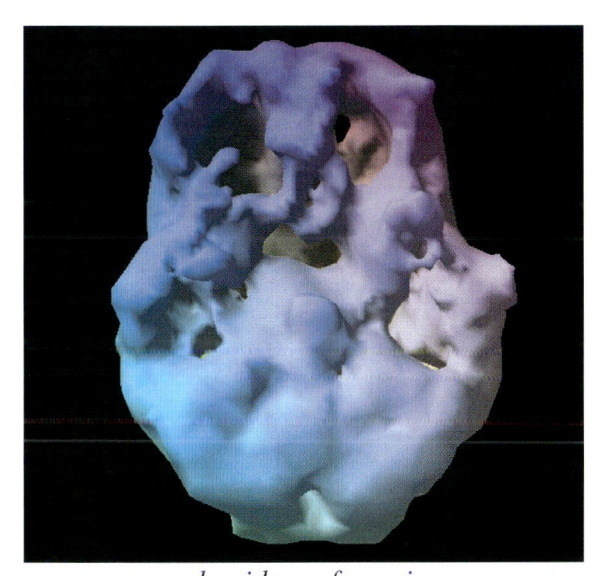

underside surface view
during substance abuse

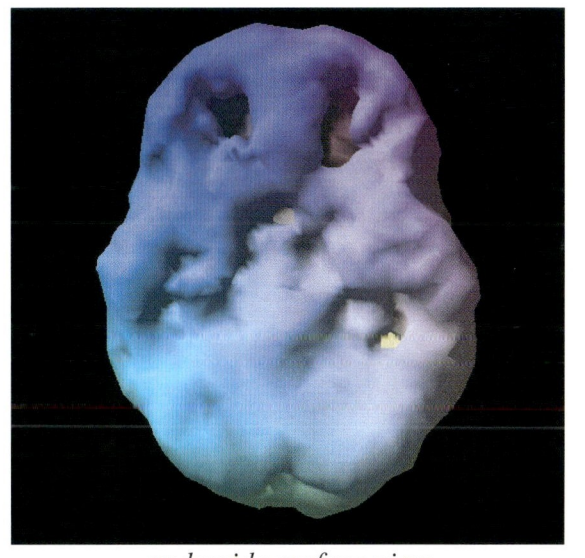

underside surface view
a year drug and alcohol free

notice the overall holes and shriveled appearance during abuse and marked improvement with abstinence

Images of Alcohol and Drug Abuse

SECTION 16

Images of Treatment

Hope for Healing

This is perhaps the most important section of this atlas. It shows actual images of treatment, the before and after SPECT images of our patients who have experienced significant benefit from treatment. This section highlights that in many cases the brain can be healed or optimized to produce greater function and subsequently a healthier, happier life.

The opening case history is one that was listed in a previous section. It is such an important and instructive case study that it warrants repeating.

A 35-year-old man who had been living on the street was brought for evaluation by his mother. He had previously been diagnosed on many occassions with paranoid schizophrenia, but refused medication. His SPECT study revealed marked overall decreased activity throughout the cerebral cortex. Being able to see his own brain activity, represented by the 3D surface SPECT study above, was helpful for him. He agreed to take his medication under his mother's supervision. One month later, after significant clinical improvement on 4 mg of risperidone a day a repeat SPECT study was performed which showed improved overall cerebral perfusion. Being able to see the before and after SPECT studies side by side on the imaging computer monitor again was very encouraging to the patient and helped significantly with compliance.

Paranoid Schizophrenia
Before and After Risperdal

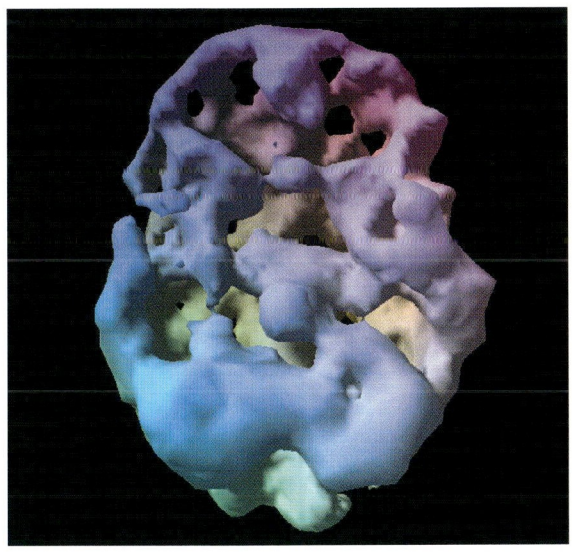

underside surface view, NO MEDS
very poor overall activity

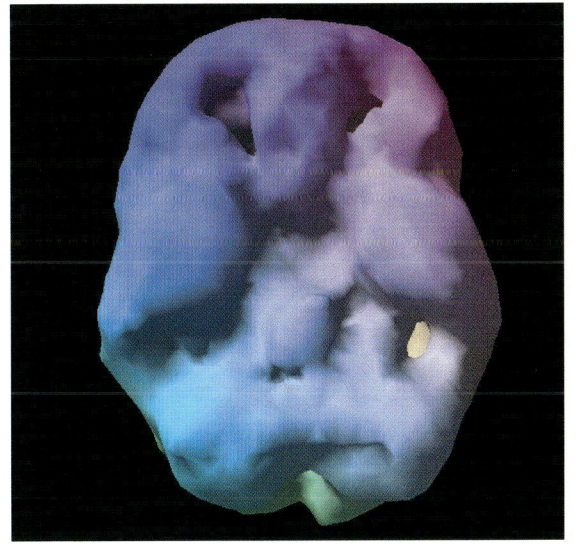

underside surface view, W/MEDS
marked overall improvement

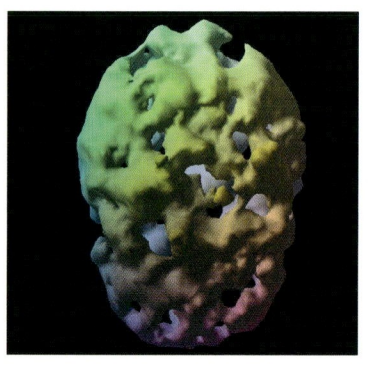

top down surface view, NO MEDS
very poor overall activity

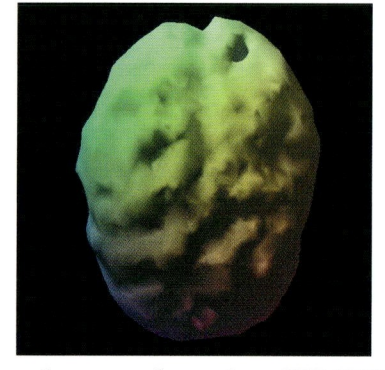

top down surface view, W/MEDS
marked overall improvement

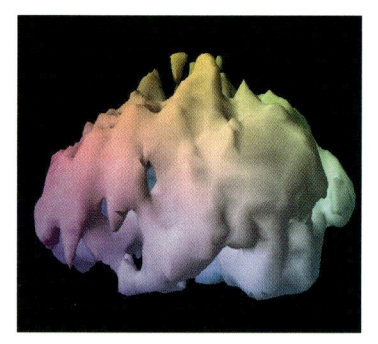

left side surface view, NO MEDS
very poor overall activity

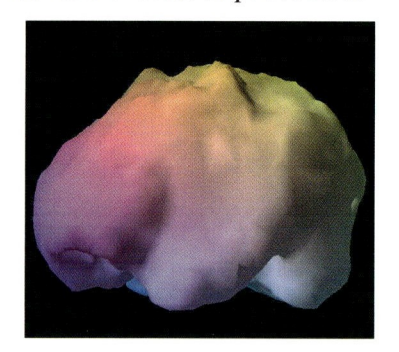

left side surface view, W/MEDS
marked overall improvement

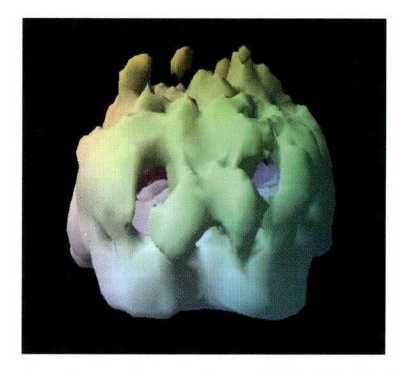

back surface view, NO MEDS
very poor overall activity

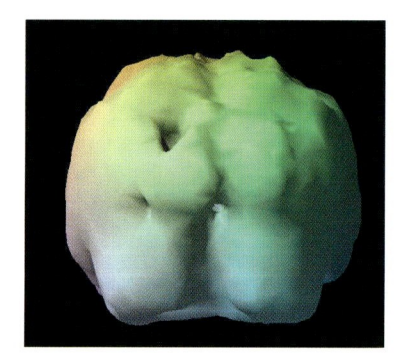

back surface view, W/MEDS
marked overall improvement

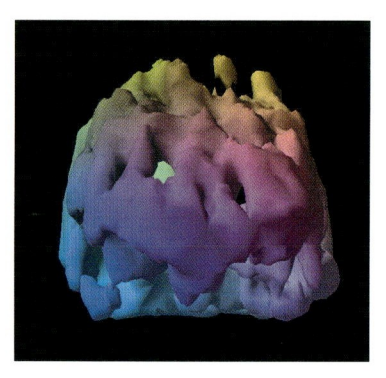

front-on surface view, NO MEDS

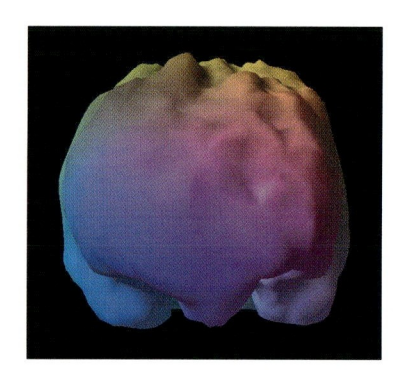

front-on surface view, W/MEDS

Images of Treatment

Suicidal, Rage
Before and After Anafranil

Bob, a 48-year-old married system analyst, came to see me because he had problems holding grudges, "getting stuck" into loops of negative thinking patterns, obsessive thoughts, moodiness, irritability, periodic intense suicidal thoughts and problems with anger control. "I am the anger broker of the valley," he reported during the initial session. His wife also reported episodes where Bob would often become upset about something, be unable to shift away from the thoughts that were upsetting him, lose control and exhibit aggressive behavior such as breaking furniture or putting holes in the walls. Bob had a childhood history of oppositional behavior (by the report of his mother). As part of his evaluation a brain SPECT study done, which showed marked increased uptake in his cingulate gyrus. I started him on Anafranil (clomipramine), which has been used in patients with obsessive thinking. Over two months of treatment the dose of Anafranil was increased to 225 mg a day. Bob and his family noted a marked positive response. He was less irritable, markedly less aggressive, more flexible and happier. He reported that he was more effective in interpersonal relationships, especially with his children.

After three years of continued clinical improvement on the same dose of clomipramine (2 brief trials at lowering the dosage caused a resumption of symptoms) a follow up brain SPECT study was ordered to evaluate brain activity subsequent to treatment. The follow-up SPECT study revealed a marked normalization of brain activity.

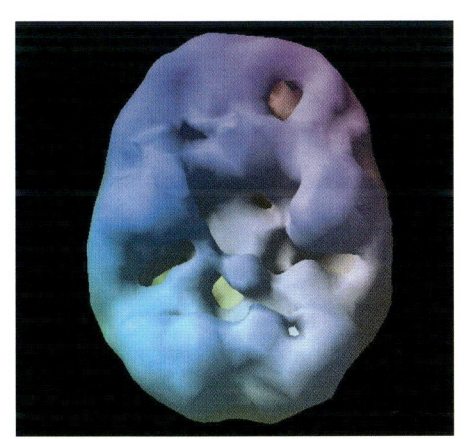

underside surface view, NO MEDS
very poor pfc/temp lobe activity

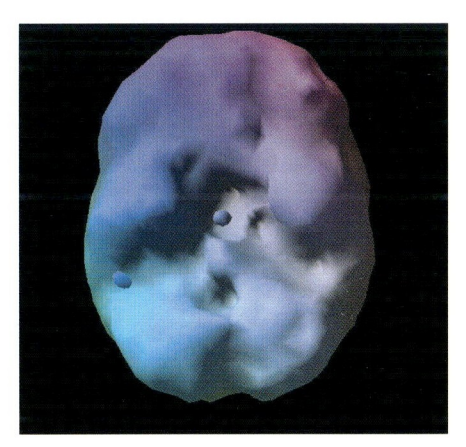

underside surface view, W/MEDS
normalization of activity

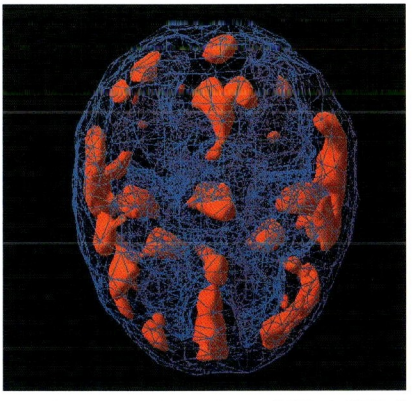

top-down active view, NO MEDS
marked increased cingulate and
left temporal lobe activity

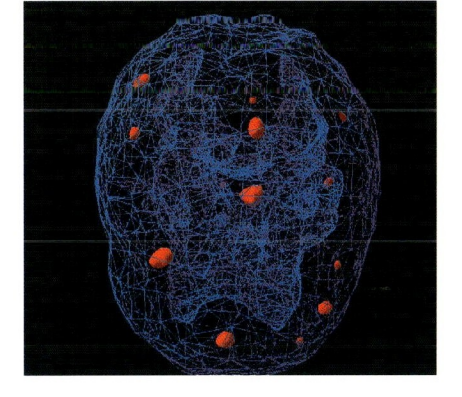

top-down active view, W/MEDS
overall improved activity

Anger, ADD

Before and After Depakote and Adderall

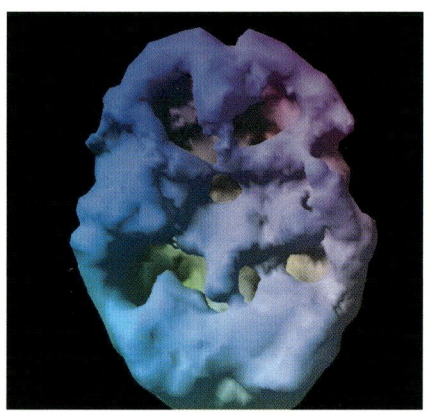

underside surface view, NO MEDS
very poor pfc/temp lobe activity

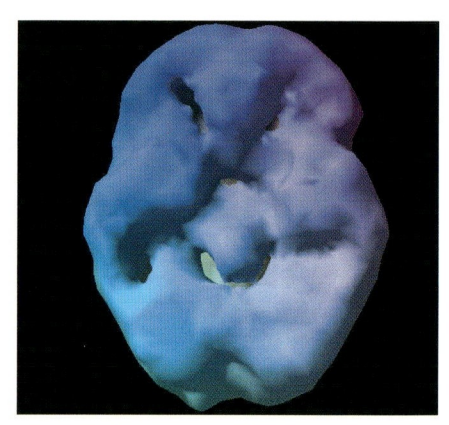

underside surface view, W/MEDS
normalization of activity

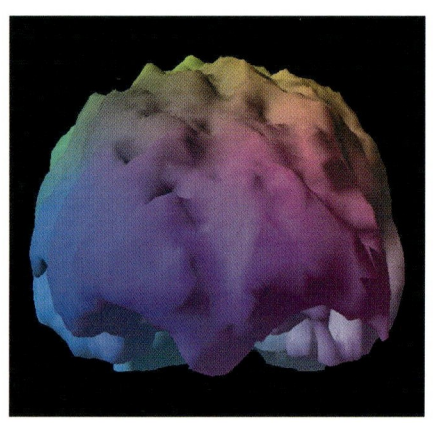

front on surface view, NO MEDS
overall scalloping of activity

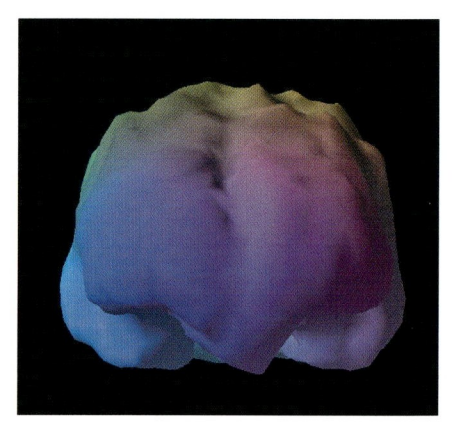

front on surface view, W/MEDS
overall improved activity

Mark, a 52-year-old married accountant, sought help for problems with concentration, focus, follow through and severe temper problems. He had become physically aggressive on several occassions with his wife. He tended to take things in a negative way and struggled with his memory. Often, for little reason he would explode and then feel very guilty about his behavior a short while later. He had longstanding school problems, despite getting an MBA degree. After his initial evaluation he was diagnosed with attention deficit disorder and a SPECT was ordered to rule out temporal lobe dysfunction. The SPECT study showed marked overall decreased activity, especially in the prefrontal cortex and temporal lobes. He was placed on a combination of Adderall (for ADD) and Depakote (for temper). He had a very positive response to medication. He and his wife reported that he was more focused, better able to follow through on tasks, less irritable and in much better control of his temper. After three years of continued clinical improvement on the same dose of Depakote and Adderall a follow-up brain SPECT study was ordered to evaluate brain activity subsequent to treatment. The follow-up SPECT study revealed a marked normalization of brain activity.

IMAGES OF HUMAN BEHAVIOR

PTSD, Depression and Anxiety

Before and After St. John's Wort and EMDR

Linda was 26 years old when she first came to see me. She had a history of 2 prior violent rapes (age 15 & 22), a physically abusive love relationship, along with experiencing the deaths of 8 friends (age 14-16). Her symptoms were depression, anxiety, worry and drug use. Her baseline SPECT study showed marked overactivity in the cingulate (problems shifting attention), basal ganglia (anxiety) and limbic areas (depression and mood dyscontrol). After 4 psychotherapy sessions with EMDR (a specific treatment technique for traumatic events) and 1 month of St. John's Wort (900 milligrams a day) Linda felt significantly better. When we repeated her SPECT study there was marked normalization of activity in all 3 areas.

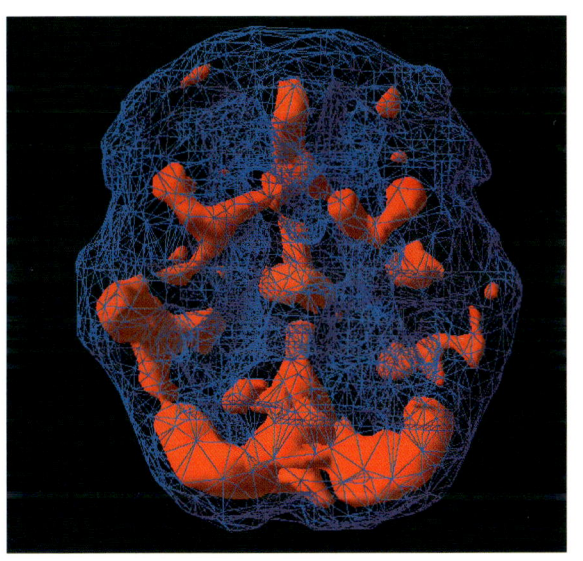

underside active view, NO MEDS

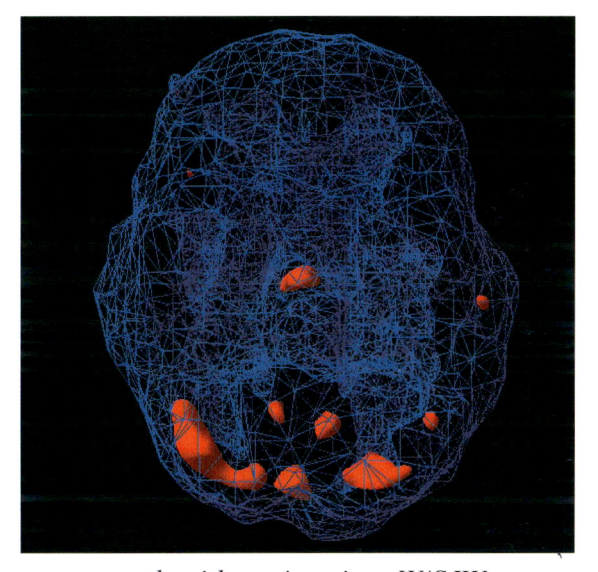

underside active view, W/SJW

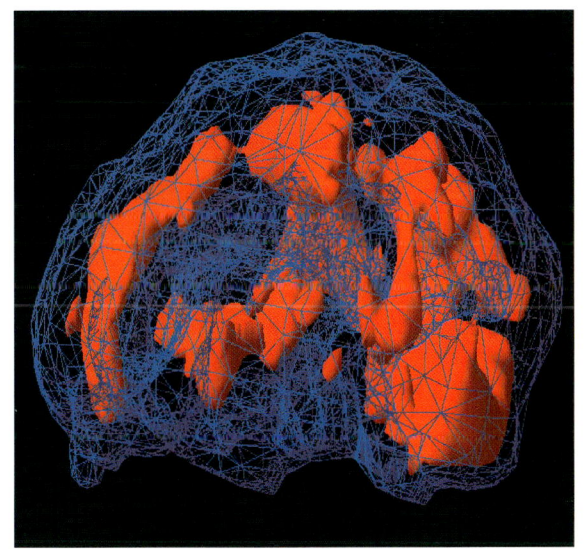

left side active view, NO MEDS marked increased cingulate, basal ganglia and limbic activity

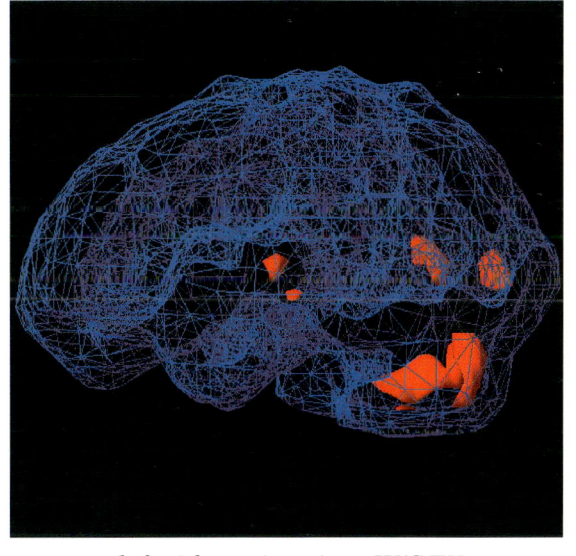

left side active view, W/SJW overall improved activity

Attention Deficit Disorder

Before and After Adderall

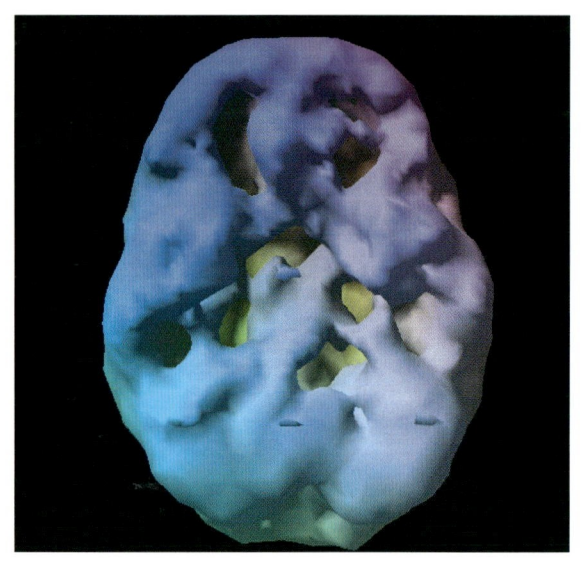

underside surface view, NO MEDS
very poor pfc and temporal lobe activity

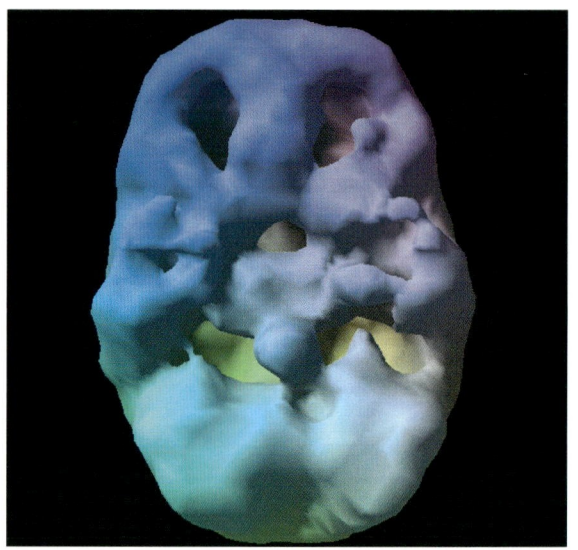

underside surface view, NO MEDS
very poor pfc and temporal lobe activity

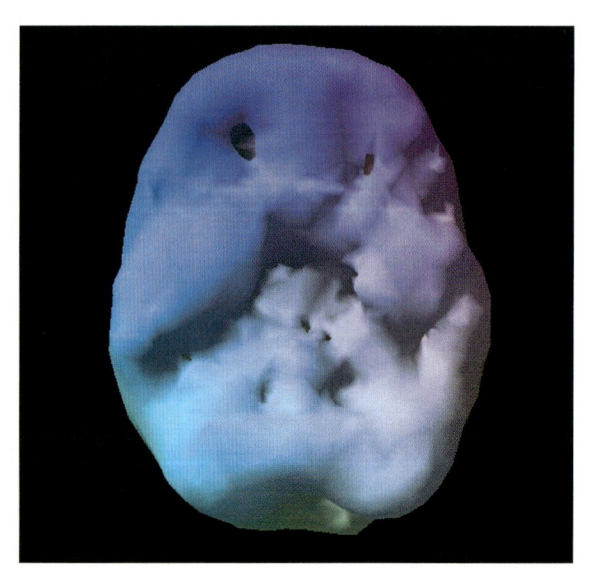

underside surface view, with Adderall
marked overall improvement

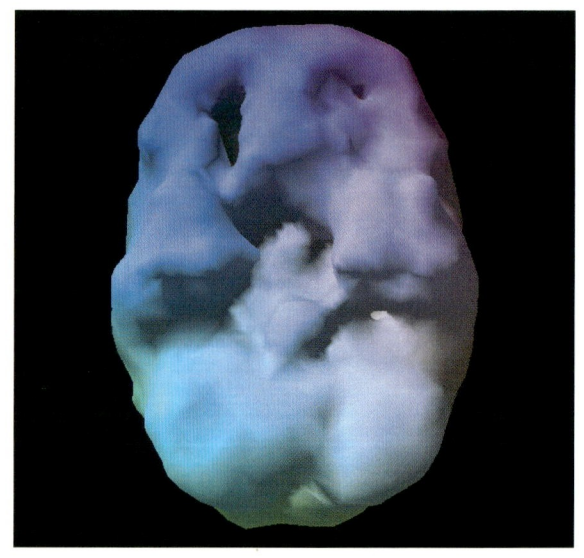

underside surface view, with Adderall
marked overall improvement

Images of Treatment

Attention Deficit Disorder

Before and After Dexedrine

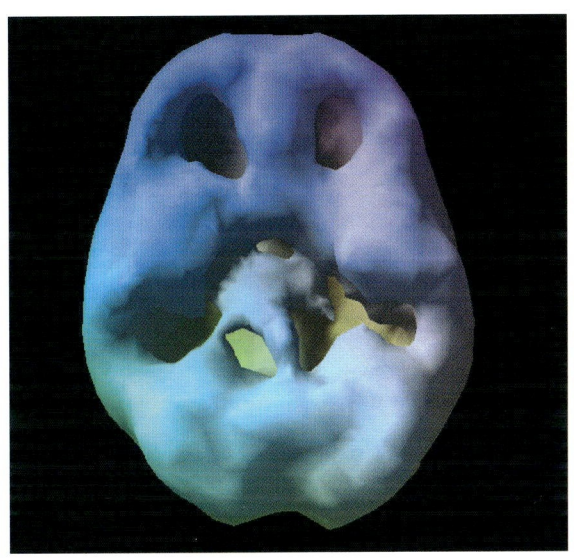

underside surface view, NO MEDS
very poor pfc and temporal lobe activity

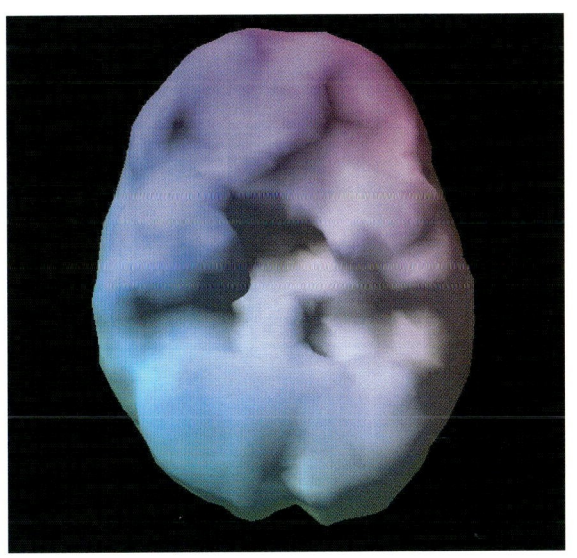

underside surface view, with Dexedrine
marked overall improvement

Conduct Disorder
Before and After carbamazepine

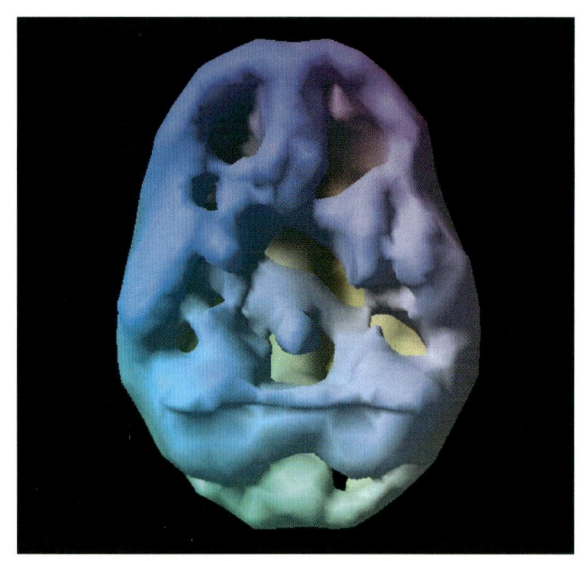

undersurface view, NO MEDS
very poor prefrontal and temporal lobe activity

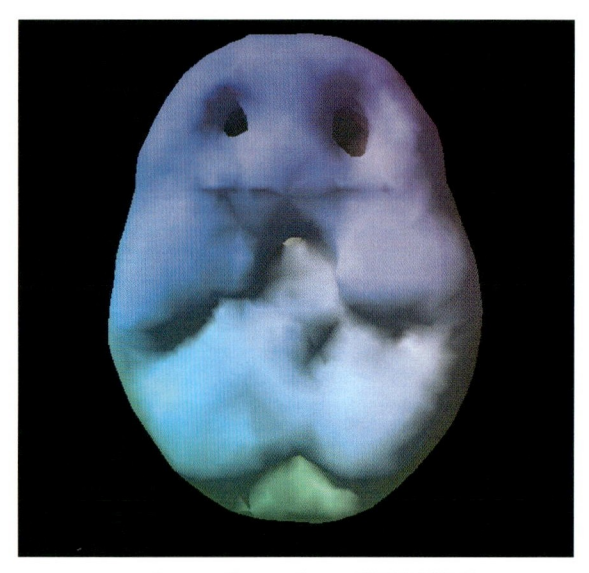

undersurface view, W/MEDS
overall improved activity

Memory, Anger, ADD

Before and After Adderall and Depakote

Russ had serious problems with unresponsive ADD symptoms, anger outbursts and memory problems. Here is his SPECT study before and 1 year after treatment with Adderall and Depakote.

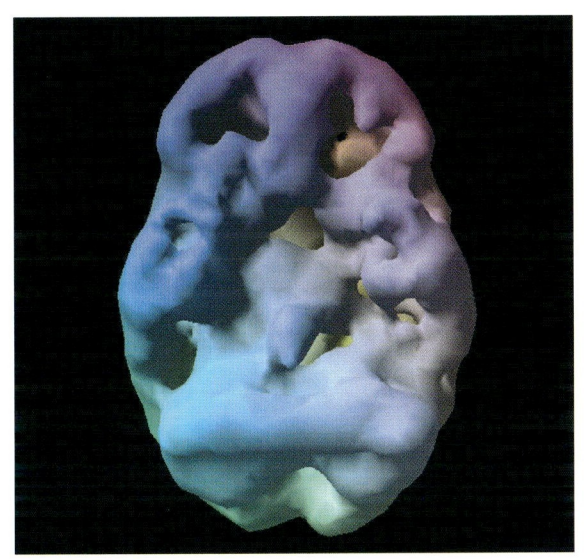

underside surface view, NO MEDS
very poor pfc/temp lobe activity

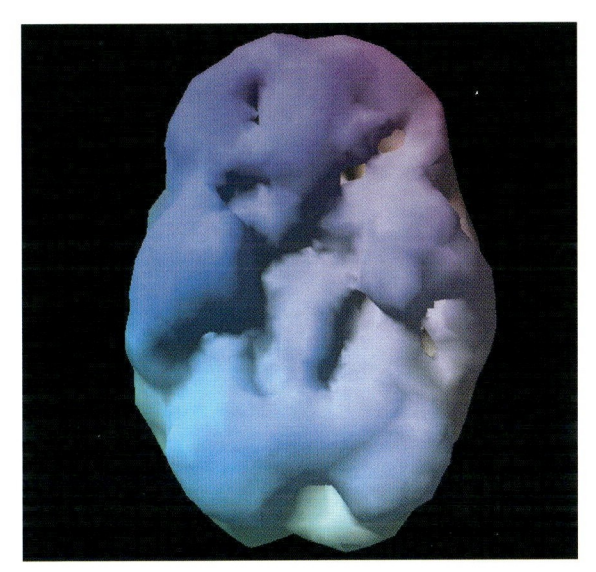

underside surface view, W/MEDS
overall improvement

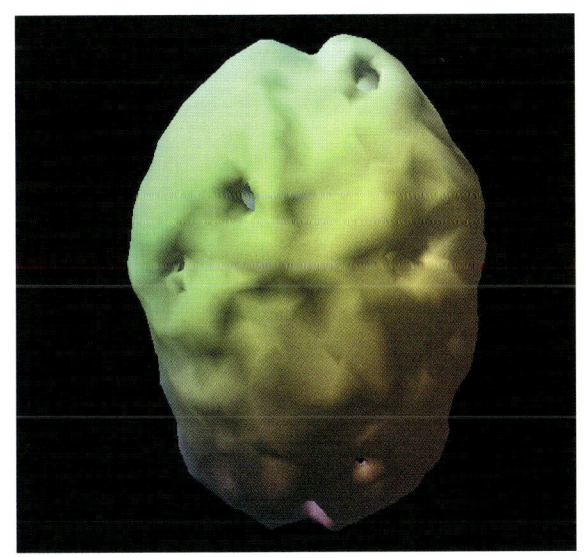

top down surface view, NO MEDS
overall decreased activity

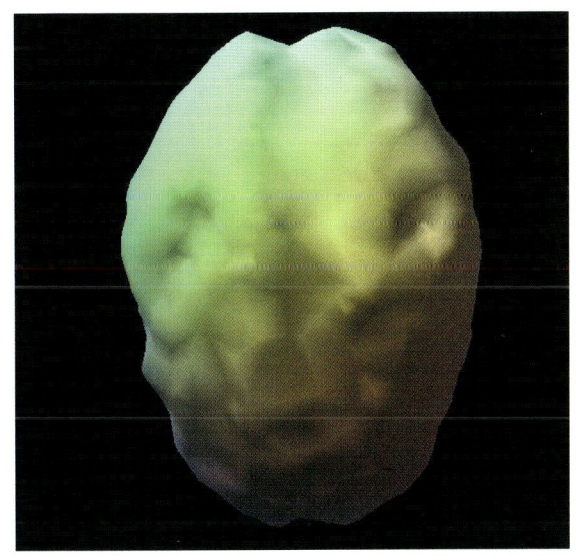

top down surface view, W/MEDS
overall improvement

Asperger's Syndrome

Before and After Zyprexa

Tim, age 12, was diagnosed with Asperger's Syndrome. He had problems with repetitive behaviors and very poor social skills. In addition, he was rigid in his thinking and had frequently temper outbursts. His baseline SPECT study revealed marked increased patchy uptake throughout his cerebral cortex. Zyprexa had an overall calming effect on his brain and significantly improved his temper and cognitive inflexibility.

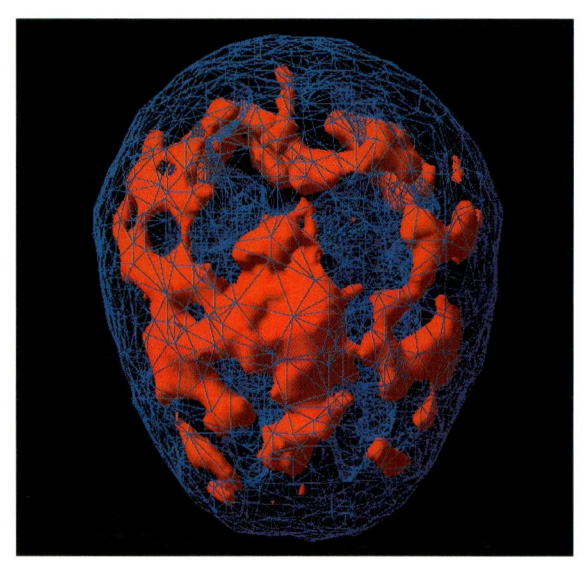

top down surface view, NO MEDS
marked patchy increased uptake

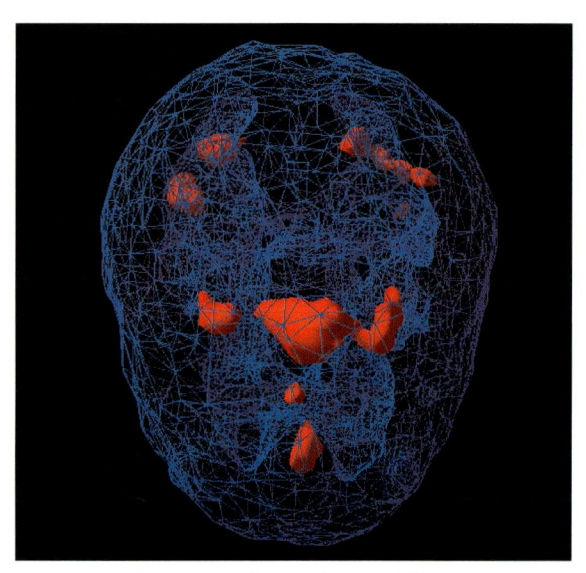

top down surface view, w/Zyprexa
overall calming effect

Severe Head Trauma

Before and After Adderall

Randy, age 17, sustained a severe blow to the left side of his head. He had a subdural bleed over his left parietal lobe and subsequently developed temper problems, school problems, speech and coordination problems. This scan series was performed on and off Adderall. Note the marked overall improvement from Adderall, giving him more access to brain function.

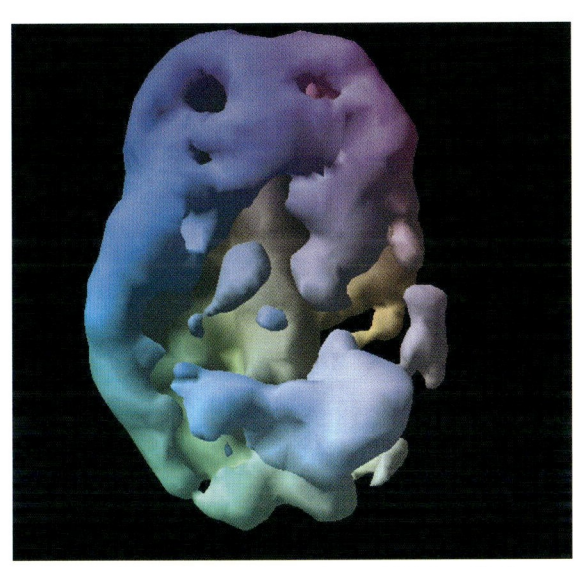

underside surface view, NO MEDS
very poor pfc and temporal lobe activity

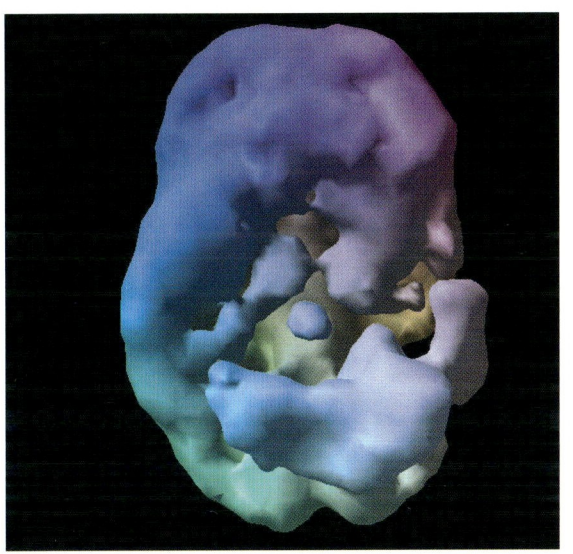

underside surface view, w/Adderall
marked overall improved activity

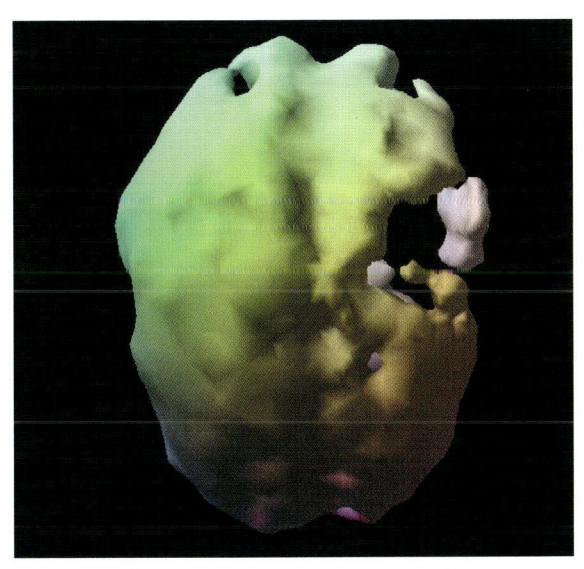

top down surface view, NO MEDS
severe decreased left parietal area

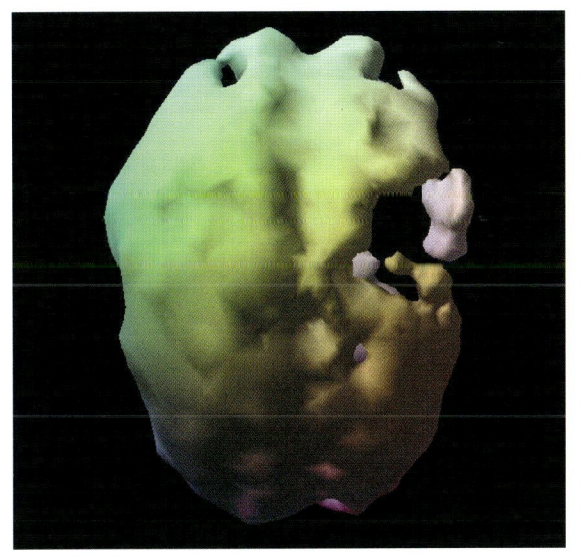

top down surface view, with Adderall
overall enhanced activity

Anger/Severe ODD

Before and After Risperdal

Mark, a 14-year-old male, was evaluated for anger outbursts and constant defiant behavior. Psychotherapy and parent training were ineffective. Depakote, Ritalin, Dexedrine and Wellbutrin were also ineffective. Prozac made him much more aggressive. A SPECT study revealed marked hyperfrontality and he was placed on Risperdal. He had a dramatic response. He was more compliant, happier and less aggressive. Two follow-up studies were performed 1 month and 6 months later, which revealed progressive calming of the hyperfrontality.

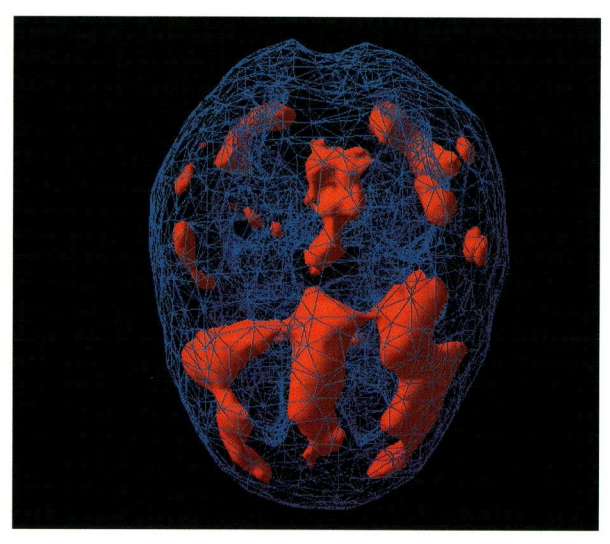

top down active view
note marked hyperfrontality

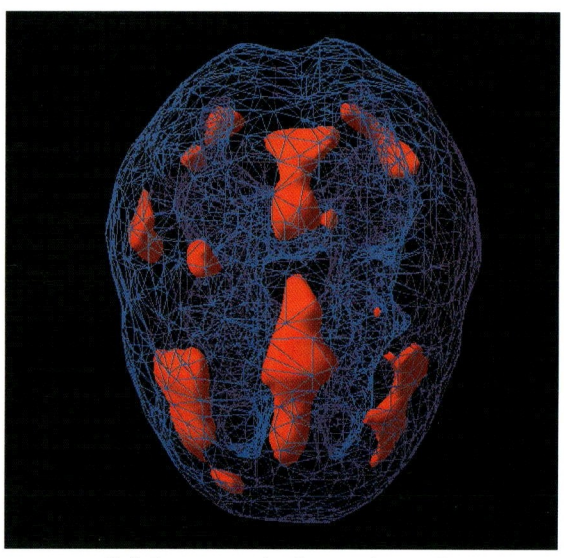

mild decrease in hyperfrontality

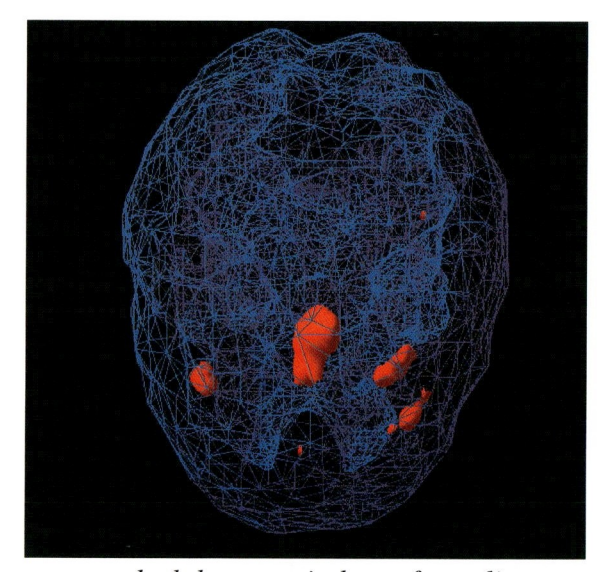

marked decrease in hyperfrontality

See www.brainplace.com for over 1250 scientific abstracts organized in the following sections:

GENERAL

NORMAL

AGGRESSION

ALCOHOL AND DRUG ABUSE

ANXIETY AND PANIC

ATTENTION DEFICIT DISORDER AND LEARNING DISABILITIES

AUTOIMMUNE DISORDER

BRAIN TRAUMA

CHRONIC FATIGUE SYNDROME

DEMENTIA / PARKINSON'S

DEPRESSION / AFFECTIVE DISORDERS

EATING DISORDERS

GILLES DE LA TOURETTE'S DISORDER

HEADACHES

INFECTIONS

MEDICATION AND OTHER TREATMENT EFFECTS

MEMORY LOSS / COGNITIVE IMPAIRMENT / DYSLEXIA

OBSESSIVE COMPULSIVE DISORDER

OCCUPATIONAL MEDICINE

SCHIZOPHRENIA

SEIZURES / PARTIAL SEIZURES

STROKE / CEREBRAL VASCULAR CHANGES

TUMORS

MISCELLANEOUS

Brain SPECT Imaging in Psychiatry/ Neurology

Bibliography

(note: only the first autor is listed to conserve save space – a full listing of the abstracts can be found at www.brainplace.com)

Books
Amen, D: Change Your Brain, Change Your Life, Random House, New York 1999

Amen, D: Healing ADD, The Breakthrough Program That Allows You to See and Heal the Six Types of Attention Deficit Disorder, GP Putnam and Sons 2/2001

Amen, D: Healing The Hardware of the Soul, Free Press, 2/2002

Book Chapters by Dr. Amen
Functional neuroimaging in clinical practice (with Joseph C. Wu and H. Stefan Bracha) in The Comprehensive Textbook of Psychiatry Edited by Kaplan and Sadock 1999

Brain SPECT Imaging and ADD in Understanding, Diagnosing, and Treating AD/HD in Children and Adolescents: An Integrative Approach. Ed Incorvaia, JA, Jason Aronson, Inc, Northvale, New Jersey, 1999, 183-196.

New Directions in the Theory, Diagnosis, and Treatment of Mental Disorders: The Use of SPECT Imaging in Everyday Clinical Practice. In The Neuropsychology of Mental Disorders. Ed Koziol, LF and Stout, CE. Charles C. Thomas, Springfield, IL 1994, 286-311.

Papers by Dr. Amen
Why Don't Psychiatrists Look At The Brain: The Case for the Greater Use of SPECT Imaging in Neuropsychiatry. Neuropsychiatry Reviews. February 2001, Vol. 2, No. 1. Pages 1, 19-21.

Brain SPECT imaging in the assessment and treatment of aggressive behavior: A putative "Reward Deficiency Syndrome (RDS)" behavioral subtype. Abstract of presentation at the First Conference on "Reward Deficiency Syndrome:" Genetic Antecedents and Clinical Pathways, San Francisco, November 12-13, 2000, in Molecular Psychiatry, Volume 6 Supplement 1, February 2001, page S7

Regional Cerebral Blood Flow In Alcohol Induced Violence: A Case Study: Journal of Psychoactive Drugs, Volume 31:4, October-December 1999.

Brain SPECT Imaging in Psychiatry. Primary Psychiatry, Vol. 5, No. 8, pgs 83-90, August 1998.

Attention Deficit Disorder: A Guide for Primary Care Physicians. Primary Psychiatry, Vol 5, No. 7, pgs 76-85, July 1998.

High Resolution Brain SPECT Imaging in Marijuana Smokers with AD/HD, Journal of Psychoactive Drugs, Volume 30, No. 2 April-June 1998 Pgs 1-13.

Visualizing the Firestorms in the Brain: An Inside Look at the Clinical and Physiological Connections between Drugs and Violence Using Brain SPECT Imaging, Journal of Psychoactive Drugs, Vol. 29 (4), 1997, 307-319

Oppositional Children Similar To OCD on SPECT: Implications for Treatment, Journal of Neurotherapy, August 1997, pgs 1-8

Three Years On Clomipramine: Before and After Brain SPECT Study, Ann Clin Psychiatry, Vol. 9, No. 2, 1997, pgs 113-116.

High Resolution Brain SPECT Imaging in Attention Deficit Hyperactivity Disorder, Ann Clin Psychiatry, Vol. 9, No. 2, 1997, pgs 81-86.

Brain SPECT Imaging In Psychiatric Practice: Advance for Radiological Professionals, Vol. 9 No. 16, August 5, 1996, pgs. 12-13

Brain SPECT Findings and Aggressiveness: Ann Clin Psychiatry, Vol. 8, No. 3, 1996, 129-137.

Brain SPECT Imaging and ADHD. J. Am. Acad. Child Adolesc. Psychiatry, 32:5, 1079-1080 (Letter), September 1993

General References

Alavi A: Studies of central nervous system disorders with single photon emission computed tomography and positron emission tomography: evolution over the past 2 decades. Semin Nucl Med 1991 Jan;21(1):58-81

Costa DC: The role of nuclear medicine in neurology and psychiatry. Curr Opin Neurol Neurosurg 1992 Dec;5(6):863-9

Devous MD Sr: Comparison of SPECT applications in neurology and psychiatry. J Clin Psychiatry 1992 Nov;53 Suppl:13-9

Friberg L: Brain mapping in thinking and language function. Acta Neurochir Suppl (Wien) 1993;56():34-9

Holman BL: Functional brain SPECT: the emergence of a powerful clinical method. J Nucl Med 1992 Oct;33(10):1888-904

Juni JE: Procedure guideline for brain perfusion SPECT using technetium-99m radiopharmaceuticals. J Nucl Med, 39(5):923-6 1998 May

Legido A: Technetium 99mTc-HMPAO SPECT in children and adolescents with neurologic disorders. J Child Neurol 1993 Jul;8(3):227-34

Messa C: Clinical brain radionuclide imaging studies. Semin Nucl Med 1995 Apr; 25(2):111-43

O'Connell RA. The role of SPECT brain imaging in assessing psychopathology in the medically ill. Gen Hosp Psychiatry 1991 Sep;13(5):305-12.

O'Connell RA. Single photon emission computed tomography (SPECT) with [123I]IMP in the differential diagnosis of psychiatric disorders. J Neuropsychiatry Clin Neurosci 1989 Spring;1(2):145-53.

O'Tuama LA: Brain single-photon emission computed tomography for behavior disorders in children. Semin Nucl Med 1993 Jul;23(3):255-64

Schlosser R: D2-receptor imaging with [123I]IBZM and single photon emission tomography in psychiatry: a survey of current status. J Neural Transm Gen Sect 1995;99(1-3):173-85.

Rodriguez G: Regional cerebral blood flow asymmetries in a group of 189 normal subjects at rest. Brain Topogr, 4(1):57-63 1991 Fall

Trzepacz PT: The relationship of SPECT scans to behavioral dysfunction in neuropsychiatric patients. Psychosomatics 1992 Winter;33(1):62-71

Van Heertum RL: Spect brain imaging in neurologic disease. Radiol Clin North Am 1993 Jul;31(4):881-907

Normal

Asenbaum S. Imaging of cerebral blood flow with technetium-99m-HMPAO and technetium-99m-ECD: a comparison. J Nucl Med 1998 Apr;39(4):613-8

Barthel H. Age-specific cerebral perfusion in 4- to 15-year-old children: a high-resolution brain SPET study using 99mTc-ECD. Eur J Nucl Med 1997 Oct;24(10):1245-

Bentourkia M. Comparison of regional cerebral blood flow and glucose metabolism in the normal brain: effect of aging. J Neurol Sci 2000 Dec 1;181(1-2):19-28

Catafau AM. Regional cerebral blood flow pattern in normal young and aged volunteers: a 99mTc-HMPAO SPET study. Eur J Nucl Med 1996 Oct;23(10):1329-37

Chiron C. Changes in regional cerebral blood flow during brain maturation in children and adolescents. J Nucl Med 1992 May;33(5):696-703

Cossu M. Regional cerebral blood flow: normal values in healthy volunteers obtained by a 32 probes xenon 133 inhalation system. Boll Soc Ital Biol Sper 1982 Jun 30;58(12):766-72

Daniel DG. Sex roles and regional cerebral blood flow. Psychiatry Res 1989 Jan; 27(1) :55-64

Deutsch G. Regional stability of cerebral blood flow measured by repeated technetium-99m-HMPAO SPECT: implications for the study of state-dependent change. J Nucl Med 1997 Jan;38(1):6-13

Eriksson L. Regional cerebral blood flow determined with single photon emission computed tomography and positron emission tomography. A comparative study. Acta Radiol Suppl 1986;369:453-5

Ernst T. Correlation of regional cerebral blood flow from perfusion MRI and spect in normal subjects. Magn Reson Imaging 1999 Apr;17(3):349-54

Globus M. Progressive age-related decrease in regional cerebral blood flow in healthy subjects. Isr J Med Sci 1985 Aug;21(8):662-5

Goto R. A comparison of Tc-99m HMPAO brain SPECT images of young and aged normal individuals. Ann Nucl Med 1998 Dec;12(6):333-9

Gur RC. Age and regional cerebral blood flow at rest and during cognitive activity. Arch Gen Psychiatry 1987 Jul;44(7):617-21

Hagstadius S. Regional cerebral blood flow characteristics and variations with age in resting normal subjects. Brain Cogn 1989 May;10(1):28-43

Houston AS. A method for assessing the significance of abnormalities in HMPO brain SPECT images. J Nucl Med 1994 Feb;35(2):239-44

Ichise M. Regional differences in technetium-99m-ECD clearance on brain SPECT in healthy subjects. J Nucl Med 1997 Aug;38(8):1253-60

Imran MB: Mean regional cerebral blood flow images of normal subjects using technetium-99m-HMPAO by automated image registration. J Nucl Med, 39(1):203-7 1998 Jan

Isaka Y. Quantitation of regional cerebral blood flow by single photon emission computed tomography of CBF-tracer combined with whole-brain CBF: a comparison between 123I-IMP and 99mTc-HMPAO in healthy volunteers]. Kaku Igaku 1994 May;31(5):423-9

Itoh M. Stability of cerebral blood flow and oxygen metabolism during normal aging. Gerontology 1990;36(1):43-8

Iwata K, Harano H. Regional cerebral blood flow changes in aging. Acta Radiol Suppl 1986;369:440-3

Jibiki I. Quantitative assessment of regional cerebral blood flow with 123I-IMP in normal adult subjects. Acta Neurol (Napoli) 1993 Feb;15(1):7-15

Jonsson C. Reproducibility and repeatability of 99Tcm-HMPAO rCBF SPET in normal subjects at rest using brain atlas matching. Nucl Med Commun 2000 Jan;21(1):9-18

Kawahata N. Reduction in mean cerebral blood flow measurements using 99mTc-ECD-SPECT during normal aging. Kaku Igaku 1997 Oct;34(10):909-16

Kawashima R. Normal cerebral perfusion of 99mTc-ECD brain SPECT—evaluation by an anatomical standardization technique. Kaku Igaku 1996 Jan;33(1):69-72

Kemp PM. Cerebral perfusion and psychometric testing in military amateur boxers and controls. J Neurol Neurosurg Psychiatry 1995 Oct;59(4):368-74

Krausz Y. Age-related changes in brain perfusion of normal subjects detected by 99mTc-HMPAO SPECT. Neuroradiology 1998 Jul;40(7):428-34

Kobayashi A. A quantitative study of regional cerebral blood flow in childhood using 123I-IMP-SPECT: with emphasis on age-related changes. No To Hattatsu 1996 Nov;28(6):501-7

Koyama M. Normal cerebral perfusion of 99mTc-HMPAO brain SPECT—evaluation by anatomical standardization technique. Kaku Igaku 1995 Sep;32(9):969-77

Koyama M. SPECT imaging of normal subjects with technetium-99m-HMPAO and technetium-99m-ECD. J Nucl Med 1997 Apr;38(4):587-92

Kuji I. Age-related changes in the cerebral distribution of 99mTc-ECD from infancy to adulthood. J Nucl Med 1999 Nov;40(11):1818-23

Lobaugh NJ: Three brain SPECT region-of-interest templates in elderly people: normative values, hemispheric asymmetries, and a comparison of single- and multihead cameras. J Nucl Med 2000 Jan;41(1):45-56

Markus HS. Alterations in regional cerebral blood flow, with increased temporal interhemispheric asymmetries, in the normal elderly: an HMPAO SPECT study. Nucl Med Commun 1993 Aug;14(8):628-33

Martin AJ. Decreases in regional cerebral blood flow with normal aging. J Cereb Blood Flow Metab 1991 Jul;11(4):684-9

Mathew RJ. Determinants of resting regional cerebral blood flow in normal subjects. Biol Psychiatry 1986 Aug;21(10):907-14

Matsuda H. Noninvasive measurements of regional cerebral blood flow using technetium-99m HMPAO. Eur J Nucl Med 1993 May;20(5):391-401

Matsuda H. Age-matched normal values and topographic maps for regional cerebral blood flow measurements by Xe-133 inhalation. Stroke 1984 Mar-Apr;15(2):336-42

Matsuda H. Age-matched normal values of regional cerebral blood flow measurements by 133Xe inhalation and production of judgment image: as to initial slope index computed by Fourier analysis. No To Shinkei 1982 Nov;34(11):1091-7

Melamed E. Reduction in rCBF during normal aging in man. Stroke 1980 Jan-Feb;11(1):31-5

Mozley PD. Effects of aging on the cerebral distribution of technetium-99m hexamethylpropylene amine oxime in healthy humans. Eur J Nucl Med 1997 Jul;24(7):754-61

Nakano S. Effects of healthy aging on the regional cerebral blood flow measurements using 99mTc-ECD SPECT assessed with statistical parametric mapping. Nippon Ronen Igakkai Zasshi 2000 Jan;37(1):49-55

Odano I. A comparative study of the quality of SPECT images obtained by 123I-IMP, 99mTc-HMPAO and 99mTc-ECD. Kaku Igaku 1997 Mar;34(3):189-94

Ogawa A. Regional cerebral blood flow with age: changes in rCBF in childhood. Neurol Res 1989 Sep;11(3):173-6

Ogawa A. Regional cerebral blood flow in children—normal value and regional distribution of cerebral blood flow in childhood. No To Shinkei 1987 Feb;39(2):113-8

Oku N. Intra-individual differences between technetium-99m-HMPAO and technetium-99m-ECD in the normal medial temporal lobe. J Nucl Med 1997 Jul;38(7):1109-11

Patterson JC. SPECT image analysis using statistical parametric mapping: comparison of technetium-99m-HMPAO and technetium-99m-ECD. J Nucl Med 1997 Nov;38(11):1721-5

Rodriguez G. Regional cerebral blood flow asymmetries in a group of 189 normal subjects at rest. Brain Topogr 1991 Fall;4(1):57-63.

Rodriguez G. Sex differences in regional cerebral blood flow. J Cereb Blood Flow Metab 1988 Dec;8(6):783-9

Schiepers C. Normal brain perfusion pattern of technetium-99m-ethylcysteinate dimer in children. J Nucl Med 1997 Jul;38(7):1115-20

Schultz SK. Age-related changes in regional cerebral blood flow among young to mid-life adults. Neuroreport 1999 Aug 20;10(12):2493-6

Schwartz RS. Regional cerebral blood flow and recognition memory in elderly normals: potential application to Alzheimer's disease. Clin Exp Neurol 1991;28:56-65

Shirahata N. Regional cerebral blood flow assessed by 133Xe inhalation and emission tomography: normal values. J Comput Assist Tomogr 1985 Sep-Oct;9(5):861-6

Slosman DO. 133Xe spect cerebral blood flow study in a healthy population: determination of t-scores. J Nucl Med 2001 Jun;42(6):864-70

Strickland TL. Cerebral perfusion and neuropsychological consequences of chronic cocaine use. J Neuropsychiatry Clin Neurosci 1993 Fall;5(4):419-27

Syed GM. Quantification of regional cerebral blood flow (rCBF) using 99Tcm-HMPAO and SPECT: choice of the reference region. Nucl Med Commun 1992 Nov;13(11):811-6

Tanaka F. Normal patterns on 99mTc-ECD brain SPECT scans in adults. J Nucl Med 2000 Sep;41(9):1456-64

Tokumaru AM. The evolution of cerebral blood flow in the developing brain: evaluation with iodine-123 iodoamphetamine SPECT and correlation with MR imaging. AJNR Am J Neuroradiol 1999 May;20(5):845-52

Vereshchagin NV. Normal values for regional cerebral blood flow using the 133Xe-inhalation method]. Zh Nevropatol Psikhiatr Im S S Korsakova 1983;83(9):1281-6

Waldemar G. 99mTc-d,l-HMPAO and SPECT of the brain in normal aging. J Cereb Blood Flow Metab 1991 May;11(3):508-21

Wirestam R. Regional cerebral blood flow distributions in normal volunteers: dynamic susceptibility contrast MRI compared with 99mTc-HMPAO SPECT. J Comput Assist Tomogr 2000 Jul-Aug;24(4):526-30

Yamashita K. Effect of smoking on regional cerebral blood flow in the normal aged volunteers. Gerontology 1988;34(4):199-204

Yang D. Normal distribution of CBF with advancing age measured by HMPAO SPECT. Nippon Igaku Hoshasen Gakkai Zasshi 1996 Oct;56(12):860-5

Aggression

Amen DG. Regional cerebral blood flow in alcohol-induced violence: a case study. J Psychoactive Drugs 1999 Oct-Dec;31(4):389-93

Amen DG. Visualizing the firestorms in the brain: an inside look at the clinical and physiological connections between drugs and violence using brain SPECT imaging. J Psychoactive Drugs 1997 Oct-Dec;29(4):307-19

Amen DG. Brain SPECT findings and aggressiveness. Ann Clin Psychiatry 1996 Sep;8(3):129-37

Barratt ES. The use of anticonvulsants in aggression and violence. Psychopharmacol Bull 1993;29(1):75-81

Bars DR. Use of visual evoked-potential studies and EEG data to classify aggressive, explosive behavior of youths. Psychiatr Serv 2001 Jan;52(1):81-6

Brennan PA. Biosocial bases of antisocial behavior: psychophysiological, neurological, and cognitive factors. Clin Psychol Rev 1997;17(6):589-604

Brennan PA. Psychophysiological protective factors for male subjects at high risk for criminal behavior. Am J Psychiatry 1997 Jun;154(6):853-5

Critchley HD. Prefrontal and medial temporal correlates of repetitive violence to self and others. Biol Psychiatry 2000 May 15;47(10):928-34

Davidson RJ. Dysfunction in the neural circuitry of emotion regulation—a possible prelude to violence. Science 2000 Jul 28;289(5479):591-4

Drexler K. Neural activity related to anger in cocaine-dependent men: a possible link to violence and relapse. Am J Addict 2000 Fall;9(4):331-9

Durand E: Legal aspects of temporal lobe epilepsy in prisoners. Rev Neurol 2001 Jan;157(1):87-8

Heinz A. In vivo association between alcohol intoxication, aggression, and serotonin transporter availability in nonhuman primates. Am J Psychiatry 1998 Aug;155(8):1023-8

Hirono N. Left frontotemporal hypoperfusion is associated with aggression in patients with dementia. Arch Neurol 2000 Jun;57(6):861-6

Intrator J. A brain imaging (single photon emission computerized tomography) study of semantic and affective processing in psychopaths. Biol Psychiatry 1997 Jul 15;42(2):96-103

Jurado MA. Psychopathy and neuropsychology of the prefrontal cortex]. Actas Luso Esp Neurol Psiquiatr Cienc Afines 1996 May-Jun;24(3):148-55

Jurado MA. Criminal behavior after orbitofrontal lesion. Actas Esp Psiquiatr 2000 Sep-Oct;28(5):337-41

Kanemoto K. Violence and epilepsy: a close relation between violence and postictal psychosis. Epilepsia 1999 Jan;40(1):107-9

Kandel E. Frontal-lobe dysfunction and antisocial behavior: a review. J Clin Psychol 1989 May; 45(3) :404-13

Kuikka JT. Abnormal structure of human striatal dopamine re-uptake sites in habitually violent alcoholic offenders: a fractal analysis. Neurosci Lett 1998 Sep 11;253(3):195-7

Krishnan KR. Brain imaging correlates. J Clin Psychiatry 1999;60 Suppl 15:50-4

Kuruoglu AC. Single photon emission computerised tomography in chronic alcoholism. Antisocial personality disorder may be associated with decreased frontal perfusion. Br J Psychiatry 1996 Sep;169(3):348-54

Lester D. Neuropsychological correlates of violence and aggression: an extension to suicidal behavior. Percept Mot Skills 1999 Oct;89(2):389-92

Lueger RJ. Frontal-lobe cognitive dysfunction in conduct disorder adolescents. J Clin Psychol 1990 Nov;46(6):696-706

Mandoki MW. Evaluation and treatment of rage in children and adolescents. Child Psychiatry Hum Dev 1992 Summer;22(4):227-35

Mayberg HS. Medical-Legal Inferences From Functional Neuroimaging Evidence. Semin Clin Neuropsychiatry 1996 Jul;1(3):195-201

Mendez MF. Pedophilia and temporal lobe disturbances. J Neuropsychiatry Clin Neurosci 2000 Winter;12(1):71-6

Pietrini P. Neural correlates of imaginal aggressive behavior assessed by positron emission tomography in healthy subjects. Am J Psychiatry 2000 Nov;157(11):1772-81

Pillmann F, Rohde A. Violence, criminal behavior, and the EEG: significance of left hemispheric focal abnormalities. J Neuropsychiatry Clin Neurosci 1999 Fall;11(4):454-7

Pincus JH. Neurologic evaluation of violent juveniles. Child Adolesc Psychiatr Clin N Am 2000 Oct;9(4):777-92

Raine A. Reduced prefrontal gray matter volume and reduced autonomic activity in antisocial personality disorder. Arch Gen Psychiatry 2000 Feb;57(2):119-27

Raine A. High autonomic arousal and electrodermal orienting at age 15 years as protective factors against criminal behavior at age 29 years. Am J Psychiatry 1995 Nov;152(11):1595-600

Raine A. Autonomic nervous system factors underlying disinhibited, antisocial, and violent behavior. Biosocial perspectives and treatment implications. Ann N Y Acad Sci 1996 Sep 20;794:46-59

Raine A. Reduced prefrontal and increased subcortical brain functioning assessed using positron emission tomography in predatory and affective murderers. Behav Sci Law 1998 Summer;16(3):319-32

Raine A. Prefrontal glucose deficits in murderers lacking psychosocial deprivation. Neuropsychiatry Neuropsychol Behav Neurol 1998 Jan;11(1):1-7

Raine A. Brain abnormalities in murderers indicated by positron emission tomography. Biol Psychiatry 1997 Sep 15;42(6):495-508

Raine A. Selective reductions in prefrontal glucose metabolism in murderers. Biol Psychiatry 1994 Sep 15;36(6):365-73

Raine A. Relationships between central and autonomic measures of arousal at age 15 years and criminality at age 24 years. Arch Gen Psychiatry 1990 Nov;47(11):1003-7

Raine A. Autonomic orienting responses in 15-year-old male subjects and criminal behavior at age 24. Am J Psychiatry 1990 Jul;147(7):933-7

Scarpa A. Psychophysiology of anger and violent behavior. Psychiatr Clin North Am 1997 Jun;20(2):375-94

Seidenwurm D. Abnormal temporal lobe metabolism in violent subjects: correlation of imaging and neuropsychiatric findings. AJNR Am J Neuroradiol 1997 Apr;18(4):625-31

Soderstrom H: Reduced regional cerebral blood flow in non-psychotic violent offenders. Psychiatry Res 2000 Feb 28;98(1):29-41

Tiihonen J. Altered striatal dopamine re-uptake site densities in habitually violent and non-violent alcoholics. Nat Med 1995 Jul;1(7):654-7

Tiihonen J: Single-photon emission tomography imaging of monoamine transporters in impulsive violent behaviour. Eur J Nucl Med, 24(10):1253-60 1997 Oct

Tonkonogy JM. Violence and temporal lobe lesion: head CT and MRI data. J Neuropsychiatry Clin Neurosci 1991 Spring;3(2):189-96

Tonkonogy JM: Hypothalamic lesions and intermittent explosive disorder. J Neuropsychiatry Clin Neurosci, 4(1):45-50 1992 Winter

Trimble MR. On some clinical implications of the ventral striatum and the extended amygdala. Investigations of aggression. Ann N Y Acad Sci 1999 Jun 29;877:638-44

Volavka J. The neurobiology of violence: an update. J Neuropsychiatry Clin Neurosci 1999 Summer;11(3):307-14

Volkow ND: Neural substrates of violent behaviour. A preliminary study with positron emission tomography. Br J Psychiatry, 151():668-73 1987 Nov

Volkow ND. Brain glucose metabolism in violent psychiatric patients: a preliminary study. Psychiatry Res 1995 Nov 10;61(4):243-53

Wong MT. Positron emission tomography in male violent offenders with schizophrenia. Psychiatry Res 1997 Feb 7;68(2-3):111-23

Wong MT. Electroencephalography, computed tomography and violence ratings of male patients in a maximum-security mental hospital. Acta Psychiatr Scand 1994 Aug;90(2):97-101

Alcohol and Drug Abuse

Amen, D: High Resolution Brain SPECT Imaging in Marijuana Smokers with AD/HD, Journal of Psychoactive Drugs, Volume 30, No. 2 April-June 1998. Pgs 1-13

Amen, D: Regional Cerebral Blood Flow In Alcohol Induced Violence: A Case Study: Journal of Psychoactive Drugs, Volume 31:4, October-December 1999

Berglund M. Normalization of regional cerebral blood flow in alcoholics during the first 7 weeks of abstinence. Acta Psychiatr Scand 1987 Feb;75(2):202-8

Chang L. Effect of ecstasy [3,4-methylenedioxymethamphetamine (MDMA)] on cerebral blood flow: a co-registered SPECT and MRI study. Psychiatry Res 2000 Feb 28;98(1):15-28

Dam M. Regional cerebral blood flow changes in patients with cirrhosis assessed with 99mTc-HM-PAO single-photon emission computed tomography: effect of liver transplantation. J Hepatol 1998 Jul;29(1):78-84

Danos P. Pathological regional cerebral blood flow in opiate-dependent patients during withdrawal: a HMPAO-SPECT study. Neuropsychobiology 1998;37(4):194-9

Drexler K. Neural activity related to anger in cocaine-dependent men: a possible link to violence and relapse. Am J Addict 2000 Fall;9(4):331-9

Dupont RM. Single photon emission computed tomography with iodoamphetamine-123 and neuropsychological studies in long-term abstinent alcoholics. Psychiatry Res 1996 Jul 31;67(2):99-111

Erbas B. Regional cerebral blood flow changes in chronic alcoholism using Tc-99m HMPAO SPECT. Comparison with CT parameters. Clin Nucl Med 1992 Feb;17(2):123-7

Ernst T. Cerebral perfusion abnormalities in abstinent cocaine abusers: a perfusion MRI and SPECT study. Psychiatry Res 2000 Aug 28;99(2):63-74

Gamma A. No difference in brain activation during cognitive performance between ecstasy (3,4-methylenedioxymethamphetamine) users and control subjects: a [H2(15)O]-positron emission tomography study. J Clin Psychopharmacol 2001 Feb;21(1):66-71

Gansler DA. Hypoperfusion of inferior frontal brain regions in abstinent alcoholics: a pilot SPECT study.

George MS. Multiple previous alcohol detoxifications are associated with decreased medial temporal and paralimbic function in the postwithdrawal period. Alcohol Clin Exp Res 1999 Jun;23(6):1077-84

Gerra G. Regional cerebral blood flow and comorbid diagnosis in abstinent opioid addicts. Psychiatry Res 1998 Aug 26;83(2):117-26

Gollub RL: Cocaine decreases cortical cerebral blood flow but does not obscure regional activation in functional magnetic resonance imaging in human subjects. J Cereb Blood Flow Metab, 18(7):724-34 1998 Jul

Günther W: Functional EEG mapping and SPECT in detoxified male alcoholics. Eur Arch Psychiatry Clin Neurosci, 247(3):128-36 1997

Harris GJ. Hypoperfusion of the cerebellum and aging effects on cerebral cortex blood flow in abstinent alcoholics: a SPECT study. Alcohol Clin Exp Res 1999 Jul;23(7):1219-27

Hata T: Three-dimensional mapping of local cerebral perfusion in alcoholic encephalopathy with and without Wernicke-Korsakoff syndrome. J Cereb Blood Flow Metab, 7(1):35-44 1987 Feb

Hermle L. Blood flow and cerebral laterality in the mescaline model of psychosis. Pharmacopsychiatry 1998 Jul;31 Suppl 2:85-91

Herning RI. The regulation of cerebral blood flow during intravenous cocaine administration in cocaine abusers. Ann N Y Acad Sci 1999;890:489-94

Holman BL. Brain perfusion is abnormal in cocaine-dependent polydrug users: a study using technetium-99m-HMPAO and SPECT. J Nucl Med, 32(6):1206-10 1991 Jun

Holman BL: A comparison of brain perfusion SPECT in cocaine abuse and AIDS dementia complex. J Nucl Med, 33(7):1312-5 1992 Jul

Holman BL. Regional cerebral blood flow improves with treatment in chronic cocaine polydrug users. J Nucl Med 1993 May;34(5):723-7

Hunter R. The pattern of function-related regional cerebral blood flow investigated by single photon emission tomography with 99mTc-HMPAO in patients with presenile Alzheimer's disease and Korsakoff's psychosis. Psychol Med 1989 Nov;19(4):847-55

Ishikawa Y. Abstinence improves cerebral perfusion and brain volume in alcoholic neurotoxicity without Wernicke-Korsakoff syndrome. J Cereb Blood Flow Metab 1986 Feb;6(1):86-94

Iyo M: Abnormal cerebral perfusion in chronic methamphetamine abusers: a study using 99MTc-HMPAO and SPECT. Prog Neuropsychopharmacol Biol Psychiatry, 21(5):789-96 1997 Jul

Kahn DA. Dissociated effects of amphetamine on arousal and cortical blood flow in humans. Biol Psychiatry 1989 Mar 15;25(6):755-67

Kao CH. Presentation of regional cerebral blood flow in amphetamine abusers by 99Tcm-HMPAO brain SPECT. Nucl Med Commun 1994 Feb;15(2):94-8.

Kitabayashi Y. A case study of BRON (cough suppressant) tablet dependence—its social psychiatric and biological aspects. Nihon Arukoru Yakubutsu Igakkai Zasshi 2000 Oct;35(5):295-305

Kitabayashi Y. A case report of organic solvent abuse with amotivational syndrome. Nihon Arukoru Yakubutsu Igakkai Zasshi 1999 Apr;34(2):130-

Konkol RJ. Normal high-resolution cerebral 99mTc-HMPAO SPECT scans in symptomatic neonates exposed to cocaine. J Child Neurol 1994 Jul;9(3):278-83

Kosten TR. Regional cerebral blood flow during acute and chronic abstinence from combined cocaine-alcohol abuse. Drug Alcohol Depend 1998 May 1;50(3):187-95

Kucuk NO. Brain SPECT findings in long-term inhalant abuse. Nucl Med Commun 2000 Aug;21(8):769-73

Kuikka JT. Abnormal structure of human striatal dopamine re-uptake sites in habitually violent alcoholic offenders: a fractal analysis. Neurosci Lett 1998 Sep 11;253(3):195-7

Kuruoİglu AC: Single photon emission computerised tomography in chronic alcoholism. Antisocial personality disorder may be associated with decreased frontal perfusion. Br J Psychiatry, 169(3):348-54 1996 Sep

Lang CJ. The use of neuroimaging techniques for clinical detection of neurotoxicity: a review. Neurotoxicology 2000 Oct;21(5):847-55

Levin JM. Improved regional cerebral blood flow in chronic cocaine polydrug users treated with buprenorphine. J Nucl Med 1995 Jul;36(7):1211-5

Levin JM: Gender differences in cerebral perfusion in cocaine abuse: technetium-99m-HMPAO SPECT study of drug-abusing women. J Nucl Med, 35(12):1902-9 1994 Dec

Mampunza S: Cerebral blood flow in just detoxified alcohol dependent patients. A 99 m Tc-HMPAO-SPECT study. Acta Neurol Belg, 95(3):164-9 1995

Martin PR: Regional cerebral glucose utilization in chronic organic mental disorders associated with alcoholism. J Neuropsychiatry Clin Neurosci, 4(2):159-67 1992 Spring

Mathew RJ. Caffeine and cerebral blood flow. Br J Psychiatry 1983 Dec;143:604-8

Mathew RJ. Dextroamphetamine-induced changes in regional cerebral blood flow. Psychopharmacology (Berl) 1985;87(3):298-302

Mathew RJ. Regional cerebral blood flow changes associated with ethanol intoxication. Stroke 1986 Nov-Dec;17(6):1156-9

Mathew RJ. Regional cerebral blood flow changes associated with amyl nitrite inhalation. Br J Addict 1989 Mar;84(3):293-99

Mathew RJ. Acute changes in cerebral blood flow associated with marijuana smoking. Acta Psychiatr Scand 1989 Feb;79(2):118-28

Mathew RJ. Acute changes in cerebral blood flow after smoking marijuana. Life Sci 1993;52(8):757-

Mathew RJ. Changes in middle cerebral artery velocity after marijuana. Biol Psychiatry 1992 Jul 15;32(2):164-9

Mathew RJ. Middle cerebral artery velocity during upright posture after marijuana smoking. Acta Psychiatr Scand 1992 Aug;86(2):173-8

Mathew RJ. Regional cerebral blood flow after marijuana smoking. J Cereb Blood Flow Metab 1992 Sep;12(5):750-8

Mathew RJ: Substance abuse and cerebral blood flow. Am J Psychiatry, 148(3):292-305 1991 Mar

Mathew RJ. Acute changes in cranial blood flow after cocaine hydrochloride. Biol Psychiatry 1996 Oct 1;40(7):609-16

Mathew RJ. Changes in cerebral blood velocity after intravenous diazepam. Biol Psychiatry 1992 Apr 1;31(7):690-7

Mathew RJ. Marijuana intoxication and brain activation in marijuana smokers. Life Sci 1997;60(23):2075-89

McCann UD. Cognitive performance in (+/-) 3,4-methylenedioxymethamphetamine (MDMA, "ecstasy") users: a controlled study. Psychopharmacology (Berl) 1999 Apr;143(4):417-25

Melgaard B. Regional cerebral blood flow in chronic alcoholics measured by single photon emission computerized tomography. Acta Neurol Scand 1990 Aug;82(2):87-93

Mena I. Cerebral blood flow changes with acute cocaine intoxication: clinical correlations with SPECT, CT, and MRI. NIDA Res Monogr 1994;138():161-73.

Mendelson JH: Improved regional cerebral blood flow in chronic cocaine polydrug users treated with buprenorphine. J Nucl Med 1995 Jul;36(7):1211-5

Miller BL: Neuropsychiatric effects of cocaine: SPECT measurements. J Addict Dis, 11(4):47-58 1992

Modell JG, Mountz JM. Focal cerebral blood flow change during craving for alcohol measured by SPECT. J Neuropsychiatry Clin Neurosci 1995 Winter;7(1):15-22

Nicolas JM. Regional cerebral blood flow-SPECT in chronic alcoholism: relation to neuropsychological testing. J Nucl Med 1993 Sep;34(9):1452-9

O'Carroll R. Neuropsychological and neuroimaging aspects of latent hepatic encephalopathy (LHE). Alcohol Alcohol Suppl 1993;2:191-5

Okada S. Regional cerebral blood flow abnormalities in chronic solvent abusers. Psychiatry Clin Neurosci 1999 Jun;53(3):351-6

O'Leary DS. Acute marijuana effects on rCBF and cognition: a PET study. Neuroreport 2000 Nov 27;11(17):3835-41

Ricaurte GA. Toxicodynamics and long-term toxicity of the recreational drug, MDMA, 'Ecstasy'. Toxicol Lett 2000 Mar 15;112-113:143-6

Riikonen R. Brain perfusion SPECT and MRI in fetal alcohol syndrome. Dev Med Child Neurol 1999 Oct;41(10):652-9

Rose JS: Cerebral perfusion in early and late opiate withdrawal: a technetium-99m-HMPAO SPECT study. Psychiatry Res, 96(1):39-47 1996 May 31

Ryu YH. Cerebral perfusion impairment in a patient with toluene abuse. J Nucl Med 1998 Apr;39(4):632-3

Sano M. Acute effects of alcohol on regional cerebral blood flow in man. J Stud Alcohol 1993 May;54(3):369-76

Schwartz JA: Acute effects of alcohol administration on regional cerebral blood flow: the role of acetate. Alcohol Clin Exp Res 1993 Dec;17(6):1119-23

Semple WE: Attention and regional cerebral blood flow in posttraumatic stress disorder patients with substance abuse histories. Psychiatry Res, 67(1):17-28 1996 May 31

Semple WE. Higher brain blood flow at amygdala and lower frontal cortex blood flow in PTSD patients with comorbid cocaine and alcohol abuse compared with normals. Psychiatry 2000 Spring;63(1):65-74

Shih WJ: Volume and surface three-dimensional displays of Tc-99m HMPAO brain SPECT imaging in a chronic hypnosedative abuser. Clin Nucl Med 1993 Jun;18(6):506-9

Strickland TL: Cerebral perfusion and neuropsychological consequences of chronic cocaine use. J Neuropsychiatry Clin Neurosci 1993 Fall;5(4):419-27

Tumeh SS. Cerebral abnormalities in cocaine abusers: demonstration by SPECT perfusion brain scintigraphy. Radiology, 176(3):821-4 1990 Sep

Tunving K: Regional cerebral blood flow in long-term heavy cannabis use. Psychiatry Res, 17(1):15-21 1986 Jan

Tutus A. Transient frontal hypoperfusion in Tc-99m HMPAO SPECT imaging during alcohol withdrawal. Biol Psychiatry 1998 Jun 15;43(12):923-8

van de Bor M. Increased cerebral blood flow velocity in infants of mothers who abuse cocaine. Pediatrics 1990 May;85(5):733-6

van Dyck CH. SPECT regional cerebral blood flow alterations in naltrexone-precipitated withdrawal from buprenorphine. Psychiatry Res 1994 Dec;55(4):181-91

Volkow ND: Brain glucose metabolism in chronic marijuana users at baseline and during marijuana intoxication. Psychiatry Res, 67(1):29-38 1996 May 31

Volkow ND: Long-term frontal brain metabolic changes in cocaine abusers. Synapse, 11(3):184-90 1992 Jul

Volkow ND. Cerebral blood flow in chronic cocaine users: a study with positron emission tomography. Br J Psychiatry 1988 May;152:641-8

Volkow ND. Association of methylphenidate-induced craving with changes in right striato-orbitofrontal metabolism in cocaine abusers: implications in addiction. Am J Psychiatry 1999 Jan;156(1):19-26

Volkow ND. Imaging studies on the role of dopamine in cocaine reinforcement and addiction in humans. J Psychopharmacol 1999 Dec;13(4):337-45

Volkow ND. Enhanced sensitivity to benzodiazepines in active cocaine-abusing subjects: a PET study. Am J Psychiatry 1998 Feb;155(2):200-6 Medical

Volkow ND. Cocaine abusers show a blunted response to alcohol intoxication in limbic brain regions. Life Sci 2000 Feb 11;66(12):PL161-7

Volkow ND. Recovery of brain glucose metabolism in detoxified alcoholics. Am J Psychiatry 1994 Feb;151(2):178-83

Volkow ND. Decreased brain metabolism in neurologically intact healthy alcoholics. Am J Psychiatry 1992 Aug;149(8):1016-22 Medical

Wallace EA. Acute cocaine effects on absolute cerebral blood flow. Psychopharmacology (Berl) 1996 Nov;128(1):17-20

Wang GJ: Brain imaging of an alcoholic with MRI, SPECT, and PET. Am J Physiol Imaging, 7(3-4):194-8 1992 Jul-Dec

Wang GJ. Regional brain metabolic activation during craving elicited by recall of previous drug experiences. Life Sci 1999;64(9):775-84

Wang GJ. Regional cerebral metabolism in female alcoholics of moderate severity does not differ from that of controls. Alcohol Clin Exp Res 1998 Nov;22(8):1850-4

Weber DA: SPECT and planar brain imaging in crack abuse: iodine-123-iodoamphetamine uptake and localization. J Nucl Med, 34(6):899-907 1993 Jun

Wexler BE. Functional magnetic resonance imaging of cocaine craving. Am J Psychiatry 2001 Jan;158(1):86-95

Wilson W. Brain morphological changes and early marijuana use: a magnetic resonance and positron emission tomography study. J Addict Dis 2000;19(1):1-22

Woods SW. SPECT regional cerebral blood flow and neuropsychological testing in non-demented HIV-positive drug abusers: preliminary results. Prog Neuropsychopharmacol Biol Psychiatry 1991;15(5):649-62

Anxiety/Panic

Benkelfat C: Functional neuroanatomy of CCK4-induced anxiety in normal healthy volunteers. Am J Psychiatry 1995 Aug;152(8):1180-4

De Cristofaro MT: Brain perfusion abnormalities in drug-naive, lactate-sensitive panic patients: a SPECT study. Biol Psychiatry 1993 Apr 1;33(7):505-12

Fredrikson M: Regional cerebral blood flow during experimental phobic fear. Pychophysiology 1993 Jan;30(1):126-30

Fredrikson M: Functional neuroanatomy of visually elicited simple phobic fear: additional data and theoretical analysis. Psychophysiology 1995 Jan;32(1):43-8

Gottschalk LA: The effect of anxiety and hostility in silent mentation on localized cerebral glucose metabolism. Compr Psychiatry 1992 Jan-Feb;33(1):52-9

Lucey JV. Brain blood flow in anxiety disorders. OCD, panic disorder with agoraphobia, and post-traumatic stress disorder on 99mTcHMPAO single photon emission tomography (SPET). Br J Psychiatry, 171():346-50 1997 Oct

Woods SW: Regional cerebral blood flow imaging with SPECT in psychiatric disease: focus on schizophrenia, anxiety disorders, and substance abuse. J Clin Psychiatry 1992 Nov;53 Suppl:20-5

Zohar J: Anxiety and cerebral blood flow during behavioral challenge. Dissociation of central from peripheral and subjective measures. Arch Gen Psychiatry 1989 Jun;46(6):505-10

Attention Deficit Disorder and Learning Disabilities

Amen, DG: Evaluating ADHD with Brain SPECT Imaging. (letter) J of Child and Adol Psychiatry 32:1080-1081, 1993

Horwitz B: Functional connectivity of the angular gyrus in normal reading and dyslexia. Proc Natl Acad Sci U S A, 95(15):8939-44 1998 Jul 21

Lou HC. Focal cerebral hypoperfusion in children with dysphasia and/or attention deficit isorder. Arch Neurol 1984 Aug;41(8):825-9.

Lou HC. Focal cerebral dysfunction in developmental learning disabilities. Lancet 1990 Jan 6;335(8680):8-11.

Sieg KG. SPECT brain imaging abnormalities in attention deficit hyperactivity disorder. Clin Nucl Med 1995 Jan;20(1):55-60.

Silva, F. 99mtc-Hmpao Brain Spect In Children With Attention Deficit Hyperactivity Disorder: Comparison Of Studies Before And After Treatment. The Journal of Nuclear Medicine, Proceedings of the 42nd Annual Meeting, 246P

Zametkin AJ. Cerebral glucose metabolism in adults with hyperactivity of childhood onset. N Engl J Med 1990 Nov 15;323(20):1361-6.

Ernst M: Effects of intravenous dextroamphetamine on brain metabolism in adults with attention-deficit hyperactivity disorder (ADHD). Preliminary findings. Psychopharmacol Bull 1994;30(2):219-25.

Matochik JA. Cerebral glucose metabolism in adults with attention deficit hyperactivity disorder after chronic stimulant treatment. Am J Psychiatry 1994 May;151(5):658-64.

Ernst M. Reduced brain metabolism in hyperactive girls. J Am Acad Child Adolesc Psychiatry 1994 Jul-Aug;33(6):858-68.

Matochik JA. Effects of acute stimulant medication on cerebral metabolism in adults with hyperactivity. Neuropsychopharmacology 1993 Jun;8(4):377-86.

Brain Trauma

Abdel-Dayem HM: SPECT brain perfusion abnormalities in mild or moderate traumatic brain injury. Clin Nucl Med, 23(5):309-17 1998 May

Abu-Judeh HH: Discordance between FDG uptake and technetium-99m-HMPAO brain perfusion in acute traumatic brain injury. J Nucl Med, 39(8):1357-9 1998 Aug

Abu-Judeh HH. SPET brain perfusion imaging in mild traumatic brain injury without loss of consciousness and normal computed tomography. Nucl Med Commun 1999 Jun;20(6):505-10

Adelson PD: Cerebrovascular response in infants and young children following severe traumatic brain injury: a preliminary report. Pediatr Neurosurg 1997 Apr;26(4):200-7

Alexander MJ: Regional cerebral blood flow trends in head injured patients with focal contusions and cerebral edema. Acta Neurochir Suppl 1994;60:479-81

Barclay L: Cerebral blood flow decrements in chronic head injury syndrome. Biol Psychiatry 1985; 20:146-157

Baulieu F: Technetium-99m ECD single photon emission computed tomography in brain trauma: comparison of early scintigraphic findings with long-term neuropsychological outcome. J Neuroimaging 2001 Apr;11(2):112-20

Bavetta S: A prospective study comparing SPET with MRI and CT as prognostic indicators following severe closed head injury. Nucl Med Commun 1994 Dec;15(12):961-8

Bigler ED: Neuroimaging in pediatric traumatic head injury: diagnostic considerations and relationships to neurobehavioral outcome. J Head Trauma Rehabil 1999 Aug;14(4):406-23

Bullock R. Early post-traumatic cerebral blood flow mapping: correlation with structural damage after focal injury. Acta Neurochir Suppl (Wien) 1992;55():14-7.

Cayli S: Asymptomatic or minimally symptomatic traumatic epidural haematomas: comparison of the results of surgical and conservative management related to SPECT and neuropsychological tests. Preliminary results. Neurosurg Rev 1998:21(4):226-31

Chang CC: Cerebral blood flow measurement in patients with impaired consciousness: usefulness of 99mTc-HMPAO single-photon emission tomography in clinical practice. Eur J Nucl Med 1998 Sep;25(9):1330-2

Choksey MS. 99TCm-HMPAO SPECT studies in traumatic intracerebral haematoma. J Neurol Neurosurg Psychiatry 1991 Jan;54(1):6-11

Cusumano S: Assessing brain function in post-traumatic coma by means of bit-mapped SEPs, BAEPs, CT, SPET and clinical scores. Prognostic implications. Electroencephalogr Clin Neurophysiol 1992 Nov-Dec;84(6):499-514

Ducours JL. Cranio-facial trauma and cerebral SPECT studies using N-isopropyl-iodo-amphetamine (123I). Nucl Med Commun 1990 May;11(5):361-7

Emanuelson IM: Computed tomography and single-photon emission computed tomography as diagnostic tools in acquired brain injury among children and adolescents. Dev Med Child Neurol, 39(8):502-7 1997 Aug

Eriskat J: Assessment of regional cortical blood flow following traumatic lesion of the brain. Acta Neurochir Suppl (Wien), 70():94-5 1997

Fumeya H: Analysis of MRI and SPECT in patients with acute head injury. Acta Neurochir Suppl (Wien) 1990;51:283-5

Furtak J: Epidemiology, diagnosis and prognosis in the clinical syndrome of brain concussion. Neurol Neurochir Pol 1996 Jul-Aug;30(4):625-30

Furtak J: Current views on brain concussion. Neurol Neurochir Pol, 31(2):327-34 1997 Mar-Apr

Garada B: Neuroimaging in Closed Head Injury. Semin Clin Neuropsychiatry 1997 Jul;2(3):188-195

Gilkey SJ: Cerebral blood flow in chronic posttraumatic headache. Headache 1997 Oct;37(9):583-7

Goldenberg G: Cerebral correlates of disturbed executive function and memory in survivors of severe closed head injury: a SPECT study. J Neurol Neurosurg Psychiatry 1992 May; 55(5):362-8

Goncalves JM: HM-PAO spect in head trauma. Acta Neurochir Suppl (Wien) 1992;55:11-3

Goshen E. The role of 99Tcm-HMPAO brain SPET in paediatric traumatic brain injury. Nucl Med Commun 1996 May;17(5):418-22

Gray BG. Technetium-99m-HMPAO SPECT in the evaluation of patients with a remote history of traumatic brain injury: a comparison with x-ray computed tomography. J Nucl Med 1992 Jan;33(1):52-8

Hendler T: Evidence for striatal modulation in the presence of fixed cortical injury in obsessive-compulsive disorder (OCD). Eur Neuropsychopharmacol 1999 Sep;9(5):371-6

Hofman PA. MR imaging, single-photon emission CT, and neurocognitive performance after mild traumatic brain injury. AJNR Am J Neuroradiol 2001 Mar;22(3):441-9

Ichise M. Technetium-99m-HMPAO SPECT, CT and MRI in the evaluation of patients with chronic traumatic brain injury: a correlation with neuropsychological performance. J Nucl Med 1994 Feb;35(2):217-26.

Ito H: Cerebral perfusion changes in traumatic diffuse brain injury; IMP SPECT studies. Ann Nucl Med, 11(2):167-72 1997 May

Ivanov LB. Single-photon emission computerized tomography in craniocerebral injuries in children. Khirurgiia (Mosk) 1995;(4):40-2

Jacobs A, Put E. One-year follow-up of technetium-99m-HMPAO SPECT in mild head injury. J Nucl Med 1996 Oct;37(10):1605-9

Jacobs A. Prospective evaluation of technetium-99m-HMPAO SPECT in mild and moderate traumatic brain injury. J Nucl Med 1994 Jun;35(6):942-7.

Kant R: Tc-HMPAO SPECT in persistent post-concussion syndrome after mild head injury: comparison with MRI/CT. Brain Inj, 11(2):115-24 1997 Feb

Kemp PM Cerebral perfusion and psychometric testing in military amateur boxers and controls. J Neurol Neurosurg Psychiatry 1995 Oct;59(4):368-74

Laatsch L. Incorporation of SPECT imaging in a longitudinal cognitive rehabilitation therapy programme. Brain Inj 1999 Aug;13(8):555-70

Laatsch L. Impact of cognitive rehabilitation therapy on neuropsychological impairments as measured by brain perfusion SPECT: a longitudinal study. Brain Inj 1997 Dec;11(12):851-63

Lewis DH: Functional brain imaging with cerebral perfusion SPECT in cerebrovascular disease, epilepsy, and trauma. Neurosurg Clin N Am 1997 Jul;8(3):337-44

Loutfi I: Comparison of quantitative methods for brain single photon emission computed tomography analysis in head trauma and stroke. Invest Radiol 1995 Oct;30(10):588-94

Lyczak P: Brain perfusion changes after head trauma assessed by cerebral SPECT with aminophylline test. Neurol Neurochir Pol 1998 Sep-Oct;32(5):1091-8

Maksymiuk G: Additional studies in the assessment of brain concussion Neurol Neurochir Pol 1997 May-Jun;31(3):579-85

Marion DW: Acute regional cerebral blood flow changes caused by severe head injuries. J Neurosurg 1991 Mar;74(3):407-14

Masdeu JC. Early single-photon emission computed tomography in mild head trauma. A controlled study. J Neuroimaging 1994 Oct;4(4):177-81.

Masdeu JC. Head trauma: use of SPECT. J Neuroimaging 1995 Jul;5 Suppl 1():S53-7.

Mitchener A: SPECT, CT, and MRI in head injury: acute abnormalities followed up at six months. J Neurol Neurosurg Psychiatry 1997 Jun;62(6):633-6

Nagamachi S: Regional cerebral blood flow in the patients with closed-head injury using 123I-IMP SPECT and computed tomography. Kaku Igaku 1993 Jul;30(7):707-16

Nedd K: 99mTc-HMPAO SPECT of the brain in mild to moderate traumatic brain injury patients: compared with CT—a prospective study. Brain Inj 1993 Nov-Dec;7(6):469-79

Neubauer RA: Hyperbaric oxygen for treatment of closed head injury. South Med J 1994 Sep;87(9):933-6

Neubauer RA: Cerebral oxygenation and the recoverable brain. Neurol Res 1998:20 Suppl 1():S33-6

Newton MR. A study comparing SPECT with CT and MRI after closed head injury. J Neurol Neurosurg Psychiatry 1992 Feb;55(2):92-4

Oder W: Behavioural and psychosocial sequelae of severe closed head injury and regional cerebral blood flow: a SPECT study. Journal of Neurology, Neurosurgery and Psychiatry 1992; 55:475-480

Otte A: PET and SPECT in whiplash syndrome: a new approach to a forgotten brain? J Neurol Neurosurg Psychiatry, 63(3):368-72 1997 Sep

Ozawa Y: Study of regional cerebral blood flow in experimental head injury: changes following cerebral contusion and during spreading depression. Neurol Med Chir (Tokyo) 1991 Nov;31(11):685-90

Prayer L. Cranial MR imaging and cerebral 99mTc HM-PAO-SPECT in patients with subacute or chronic severe closed head injury and normal CT examinations. Acta Radiol 1993 Nov;34(6):593-9

Reid RH: Cerebral perfusion imaging with technetium-99m HMPAO following cerebral trauma. Initial experience. Clin Nucl Med 1990 Jun;15(6):383-8

Ricker JH: Functional neuroimaging and quantitative electroencephalography in adult traumatic head injury: clinical applications and interpretive cautions. J Head Trauma Rehabil 2000 Apr;15(2):859-68

Roper SN: An analysis of cerebral blood flow in acute closed head injury using technetium-99m-HMPAO SPECT and computed tomography. J Nucl Med 1991; 32:1684-1687

Sakas DE. Focal cerebral hyperemia after focal head injury in humans: a benign phenomenon? J Neurosurg 1995 Aug;83(2):277-84.

Septien L: Value of local cerebral hypoperfusion in the diagnosis of frontal syndromes. Importance in medical expert assessment of head injuries. Encephale 1993 May-Jun;19(3):249-55

Shiina G. Sequential assessment of cerebral blood flow in diffuse brain injury by 123I-iodoamphetamine single-photon emission CT. AJNR Am J Neuroradiol 1998 Feb;19(2):297-302

Skippen P: Effect of hyperventilation on regional cerebral blood flow in head-injured children. Crit Care Med 1997 Aug;25(8):1402-9

Stepien A. Assessment of regional blood flow in patients after mild head trauma, Neurol Neurochir Pol 1999 Jan-Feb;33(1):119-29

Tokuda T: A case progressive dementia developed after repeated head trauma. 1991 Apr;31(4):468-7i

Umile EM; Plotkin RC. Functional assessment of mild traumatic brain injury using SPECT and neuropsychological testing. Brain Inj 1998 Jul;12(7):577-94

Yamakami I, Yamaura A: Types of traumatic brain injury and regional cerebral blood flow assessed by 99mTc-HMPAO SPECT. Neurol Med Chir (Tokyo) 1993 Jan;33(1):7-12.

Chronic Fatigue Syndrome

Ichise M: Assessment of regional cerebral perfusion by 99Tcm-HMPAO SPECT in chronic fatigue syndrome. Nucl Med Commun 1992 Oct;13(10):767-72

Johansson G. Cerebral dysfunction in fibromyalgia: evidence from regional cerebral blood flow measurements, otoneurological tests and cerebrospinal fluid analysis. Acta Psychiatr Scand 1995 Feb;91(2):86-94

Schwartz RB: SPECT imaging of the brain: comparison of findings in patients with chronic fatigue syndrome, AIDS dementia complex, and major unipolar depression. AJR Am J Roentgenol 1994 Apr;162(4):943-51

Dementia/Parkinson's

Alexander GE. Cortical perfusion and gray matter weight in frontal lobe dementia. J Neuropsychiatry Clin Neurosci 1995 Spring;7(2):188-96.

Arbizu J. Correlations between brain SPECT and neuropsychology assessments in mild and moderate stages of Alzheimer's disease. Rev Esp Med Nucl 1999 Aug;18(4):252-60

Arbizu J. Cerebral SPECT and neuropsychological function in Alzheimer's disease. Rev Med Univ Navarra 1997 Jan-Mar;41(1):12-8

Ashford JW. Single SPECT measures of cerebral cortical perfusion reflect time-index estimation of dementia severity in Alzheimer's disease. J Nucl Med 2000 Jan;41(1):57-64

Battistin L. Regional cerebral blood flow study with 99mTc-hexamethyl-propyleneamine oxime single photon emission computed tomography in Alzheimer's and multi-infarct dementia. Eur Neurol 1990;30(5):296-301.

Benoit M. Behavioral and psychological symptoms in Alzheimer's disease. Relation between apathy and regional cerebral perfusion. Dement Geriatr Cogn Disord 1999 Nov-Dec;10(6):511-7

Bergman H. HM-PAO SPECT brain scanning in the diagnosis of Alzheimer's disease. J Am Geriatr Soc 1997 Jan;45(1):15-20

Blanco A. Usefulness of SPECT in the study of Alzheimer's disease. Neurologia 1998 Feb;13(2):63-8

Blin J: Cholinergic neurotransmission has different effects on cerebral glucose consumption and blood flow in young normals, aged normals, and Alzheimer's disease patients. Neuroimage, 6(4):335-43 1997 Nov

Bonte FJ: Brain blood flow in the dementias: SPECT with histopathologic correlation in 54 patients. Radiology, 202(3):793-7 1997 Mar

Bonte FJ. Brain blood flow in the dementias: SPECT with histopathologic correlation. Radiology 1993 Feb;186(2):361-5

Bottino CM. Can neuroimaging techniques identify individuals at risk of developing Alzheimer's disease? Int Psychogeriatr 1997 Dec;9(4):389-403

Buchpiguel CA. Brain SPECT in dementia. A clinical-scintigraphic correlation. Arq Neuropsiquiatr 1996 Sep;54(3):375-83

Cappa A. Brain perfusion abnormalities in Alzheimer's disease: comparison between patients with focal temporal lobe dysfunction and patients with diffuse cognitive impairment. J Neurol Neurosurg Psychiatry 2001 Jan;70(1):22-7

Cardebat D. Brain correlates of memory processes in patients with dementia of Alzheimer's type: a SPECT Activation Study. J Cereb Blood Flow Metab 1998 Apr;18(4):457-62

Carroll RE. Regional cerebral blood flow and cognitive function in patients with chronic liver disease. Lancet 1991 May 25;337(8752):1250-3.

Chang L. Perfusion MRI detects rCBF abnormalities in early stages of HIV-cognitive motor complex. Neurology 2000 Jan 25;54(2):389-96

Charpentier P. Alzheimer's disease and frontotemporal dementia are differentiated by discriminant analysis applied to (99m)Tc HmPAO SPECT data. J Neurol Neurosurg Psychiatry 2000 Nov;69(5):661-3

Claus JJ. Determinants of quantitative spectral electroencephalography in early Alzheimer's disease: cognitive function, regional cerebral blood flow, and computed tomography. Dement Geriatr Cogn Disord 2000 Mar-Apr;11(2):81-9

Claus JJ. Measurement of temporal regional cerebral perfusion with single-photon emission tomography predicts rate of decline in language function and survival in early Alzheimer's disease. Eur J Nucl Med 1999 Mar;26(3):265-71

Cummings JL: Frontal lobe degeneration: clinical, neuropsychological, and SPECT characteristics [see comments] Comment in: Neurology 1992 Sep;42(9):1850-1 Arology 1991 Sep;41(9):1374-8.

Defebvre LJ. Technetium HMPAO SPECT study in dementia with Lewy bodies, Alzheimer's disease and idiopathic Parkinson's disease. J Nucl Med 1999 Jun;40(6):956-62

Demonet JF: Activation of regional cerebral blood flow by a memorization task in early Parkinson's disease patients and normal subjects. J Cereb Blood Flow Metab 1994 May;14(3):431-8

Dierckx RA. Sensitivity and specificity of 99Tcm-HMPAO single-headed SPECT in dementia. Nucl Med Commun 1993 Sep;14(9):792-7

Domper M: Brain photon emission tomography. Value of the corticocerebellar index and gammagraphic patterns in Alzheimer's disease and other diseases. Med Clin (Barc) 1991 Jan 12;96(1):1-5

Dormehl IC. SPECT monitoring of improved cerebral blood flow during long-term treatment of elderly patients with nootropic drugs. Clin Nucl Med 1999 Jan;24(1):29-34

El Fakhri G. Absolute activity quantitation in simultaneous 123I/99mTc brain SPECT. J Nucl Med 2001 Feb;42(2):300-8

Elmstahl S: A study of regional cerebral blood flow using 99mTc-HMPAO-SPECT in elderly women with senile dementia of Alzheimer's type. Dementia 1994 Nov-Dec;5(6):302-9

Engel P: Single photon emission computed tomography in dementia: relationship of perfusion to cognitive deficits. J Geriatr Psychiatry Neurol 1993 Jul-Sep;6(3):144-51

Golan H. Usefulness of follow-up regional cerebral blood flow measurements by single-photon emission computed tomography in the differential diagnosis of dementia. J Neuroimaging 1996 Jan;6(1):23-8

Hanyu H. Diagnostic accuracy of single photon emission computed tomography in Alzheimer's disease. Gerontology 1993;39(5):260-6

Hanyu H. Single photon emission computed tomography in the diagnosis of Alzheimer's disease. Nippon Ronen Igakkai Zasshi 1997 Jun;34(6):468-73

Hanyu H. Relation between Hippocampal damage and cerebral cortical function in Alzheimer's disease. Nippon Ronen Igakkai Zasshi 2000 Nov;37(11):921-7

Harris GJ. Dynamic susceptibility contrast MR imaging of regional cerebral blood volume in Alzheimer disease: a promising alternative to nuclear medicine. AJNR Am J Neuroradiol 1998 Oct;19(9):1727-32

Hellman RS. A multi-institutional study of interobserver agreement in the evaluation of dementia with rCBF/SPET technetium-99m exametazime (HMPAO). Eur J Nucl Med 1994 Apr;21(4):306-13

Herbster AN: Functional connectivity in auditory-verbal short-term memory in Alzheimer's disease. Neuroimage, 4(2):67-77 1996 Oct

Hogh P. Single photon emission computed tomography and apolipoprotein E in Alzheimer's disease: impact of the epsilon4 allele on regional cerebral blood flow. J Geriatr Psychiatry Neurol 2001 Spring;14(1):42-51

Houston AS. Use of significance image to determine patterns of cortical blood flow abnormality in pathological and at-risk groups. J Nucl Med 1998 Mar;39(3):425-30

Imran MB. Tc-99m HMPAO SPECT in the evaluation of Alzheimer's disease: correlation between neuropsychiatric evaluation and CBF images. J Neurol Neurosurg Psychiatry 1999 Feb;66(2):228-32

Imran MB. Parametric mapping of cerebral blood flow deficits in Alzheimer's disease: a SPECT study using HMPAO and image standardization technique. J Nucl Med 1999 Feb;40(2):244-9

Ishii K. Regional cerebral blood flow difference between dementia with Lewy bodies and AD. Neurology 1999 Jul 22;53(2):413-6

Jagust WJ: Cognitive function and regional cerebral blood flow in Parkinson's disease. Brain 1992 Apr;115 (Pt 2):521-37

Jagust WJ. Clinical studies of cerebral blood flow in Alzheimer's disease. Ann N Y Acad Sci 1997 Sep 26;826:254-62

Jagust WJ. Brain perfusion imaging predicts survival in Alzheimer's disease. Neurology 1998 Oct;51(4):1009-13

Jagust W: SPECT perfusion imaging in the diagnosis of Alzheimer's disease: A clinical-pathologic study. [In Process Citation] Neurology 2001 Apr 10;56(7):950-6

Jibiki I. Utility of 123I-IMP SPECT brain scans for the early detection of site-specific abnormalities in Creutzfeldt-Jakob disease (Heidenhain type): a case study. Neuropsychobiology 1994;29(3):117-9.

Jobst KA. Accurate prediction of histologically confirmed Alzheimer's disease and the differential diagnosis of dementia: the use of NINCDS-ADRDA and DSM-III-R criteria, SPECT, X-ray CT, and APO E4 medial temporal lobe dementias. Int Psychogeriatr 1997;9 Suppl 1:191-222

Jobst KA. The diagnosis of Alzheimer's disease: a question of image? J Clin Psychiatry 1994 Nov;55 Suppl:22-31

Johnson KA. Quantitative brain SPECT in Alzheimer's disease and normal aging. J Nucl Med 1993 Nov;34(11):2044-8

Johnson KA: Preclinical prediction of Alzheimer's disease using SPECT. Neurology, 50(6):1563-71 1998 Jun

Julin P: Brain volumes and regional cerebral blood flow in carriers of the Swedish Alzheimer amyloid protein mutation. Alzheimer Dis Assoc Disord, 12(1):49-53 1998 Mar

Julin P. Clinical diagnosis of frontal lobe dementia and Alzheimer's disease: relation to cerebral perfusion, brain atrophy and electroencephalography. Dementia 1995 May-Jun;6(3):142-7.

Kawabata K. Cerebral blood flow and dementia in Parkinson's disease. J Geriatr Psychiatry Neurol 1991 Oct-Dec;4(4):194-203.

Kogure D. Longitudinal evaluation of early dementia of Alzheimer type using brain perfusion SPECT. Kaku Igaku 1999 Feb;36(2):91-101

Kogure D: Longitudinal evaluation of early Alzheimer's disease using brain perfusion SPECT. J Nucl Med 2000 Jul;41(7):1155-1162.

Lavenu I. Association between medial temporal lobe atrophy on CT and parietotemporal uptake decrease on SPECT in Alzheimer's disease. J Neurol Neurosurg Psychiatry 1997 Oct;63(4):441-5

Lehtovirta M. Longitudinal SPECT study in Alzheimer's disease: relation to apolipoprotein E polymorphism. J Neurol Neurosurg Psychiatry 1998 Jun;64(6):742-6

Lenart-Jankowska D. Diagnostic value of regional cerebral blood flow in SPECT pattern in Alzheimer's disease. Neurol Neurochir Pol 1998 Sep-Oct;32(5):1023-32

Lindau M. First symptoms—frontotemporal dementia versus Alzheimer's disease. Dement Geriatr Cogn Disord 2000 Sep-Oct;11(5):286-93

Lobotesis K. Occipital hypoperfusion on SPECT in dementia with Lewy bodies but not AD. Neurology 2001 Mar 13;56(5):643-9

Masterman DL. Sensitivity, specificity, and positive predictive value of technetium 99-HMPAO SPECT in discriminating Alzheimer's disease from other dementias. J Geriatr Psychiatry Neurol 1997 Jan;10(1):15-21

Mattman A. Regional HmPAO SPECT and CT measurements in the diagnosis of Alzheimer's disease. Can J Neurol Sci 1997 Feb;24(1):22-8

Mielke R. HMPAO SPET and FDG PET in Alzheimer's disease and vascular dementia: comparison of perfusion and metabolic pattern. Eur J Nucl Med 1994 Oct;21(10):1052-60

Mori E. Role of functional brain imaging in the evaluation of vascular dementia. Alzheimer Dis Assoc Disord 1999 Oct-Dec;13 Suppl 3:S91-101

Muller H. SPECT patterns in probable Alzheimer's disease. Eur Arch Psychiatry Clin Neurosci 1999;249(4):190-6

Müller TJ: A comparison of qEEG and HMPAO-SPECT in relation to the clinical severity of Alzheimer's disease. Eur Arch Psychiatry Clin Neurosci, 247(5):259-63 1997

Nitrini R. SPECT in Alzheimer's disease: features associated with bilateral parietotemporal hypoperfusion. Acta Neurol Scand 2000 Mar;101(3):172-6

Nobler MS. Cerebral blood flow and metabolism in late-life depression and dementia. J Geriatr Psychiatry Neurol 1999 Fall;12(3):118-27

O'Brien JT. A study of regional cerebral blood flow and cognitive performance in Alzheimer's disease. J Neurol Neurosurg Psychiatry 1992 Dec;55(12):1182-7.

Okamura N. Prediction of progression in patients with mild cognitive impairment using IMP-SPECT. Nippon Ronen Igakkai Zasshi 2000 Dec;37(12):974-8

Okuda B. Comparison of brain perfusion in corticobasal degeneration and Alzheimer's disease. Dement Geriatr Cogn Disord 2001 May-Jun;12(3):226-31

Osimani A. SPECT for differential diagnosis of dementia and correlation of rCBF with cognitive impairment. Can J Neurol Sci 1994 May;21(2):104-11.

Ott BR: A single-photon emission computed tomography imaging study of driving impairment in patients with Alzheimer's disease. Dement Geriatr Cogn Disord 2000 May-Jun;11(3):153-60

Ott BR. Lateralized cortical perfusion in women with Alzheimer's disease. J Gend Specif Med 2000 Sep-Oct;3(6):29-35

Pagani M. Mapping pathological (99m)Tc HMPAO uptake in Alzheimer's disease and frontal lobe dementia with SPECT. Dement Geriatr Cogn Disord 2001 May-Jun;12(3):177-84

Passero S. Quantitative EEG mapping, regional cerebral blood flow, and neuropsychological function in Alzheimer's disease. Dementia 1995 May-Jun;6(3):148-56.

Pavics L. Regional cerebral blood flow single-photon emission tomography with 99mTc-HMPAO and the acetazolamide test in the evaluation of vascular and Alzheimer's dementia. Eur J Nucl Med 1999 Mar;26(3):239-45

Pickut BA. Discriminative use of SPECT in frontal lobe-type dementia versus (senile) dementia of the Alzheimer's type. J Nucl Med 1997 Jun;38(6):929-34

Read SL. SPECT in dementia: clinical and pathological correlation. J Am Geriatr Soc 1995 Nov;43(11):1243-7

Rodriguez G. 99mTc-HMPAO regional cerebral blood flow and quantitative electroencephalography in Alzheimer's disease: a correlative study. J Nucl Med 1999 Apr;40(4):522-9

Rodriguez G. Hippocampal perfusion in mild Alzheimer's disease. Psychiatry Res 2000 Dec 4;100(2):65-74

Sachdev P. Longitudinal study of cerebral blood flow in Alzheimer's disease using SPECT. Psychiatry Res 1997 Feb 7;68(2-3):133-41

Sackeim HA. Regional cerebral blood flow in mood disorders. II. Comparison of major depression and Alzheimer's disease. J Nucl Med 1993 Jul;34(7):1090-101.

Scheltens P. The diagnostic value of magnetic resonance imaging and technetium 99m-HMPAO single-photon-emission computed tomography for the diagnosis of Alzheimer disease in a community-dwelling elderly population. Alzheimer Dis Assoc Disord 1997 Jun;11(2):63-70

Shih WJ. Consecutive brain SPECT surface three-dimensional displays show progression of cerebral cortical abnormalities in Alzheimer's disease Clin Nucl Med 1999 Oct;24(10):773-7

Sjogren M. Frontotemporal dementia can be distinguished from Alzheimer's disease and subcortical white matter dementia by an anterior-to-posterior rCBF-SPET ratio. Dement Geriatr Cogn Disord 2000 Sep-Oct;11(5):275-85

Sloan EP. Electroencephalography and single photon emission computed tomography in dementia: a comparative study. Psychol Med 1995 May;25(3):631-8

Staff RT. Changes in the rCBF images of patients with Alzheimer's disease receiving Donepezil therapy. Nucl Med Commun 2000 Jan;21(1):37-41

Staff RT. Delusions in Alzheimer's disease: spet evidence of right hemispheric dysfunction. Cortex 1999 Sep;35(4):549-60

Staff RT. HMPAO SPECT imaging of Alzheimer's disease patients with similar content-specific autobiographic delusion: comparison using statistical parametric mapping. J Nucl Med 2000 Sep;41(9):1451-5

Starkstein SE: A single-photon emission computed tomographic study of anosognosia in Alzheimer's disease. Argentina. Arch Neurol 1995 Apr;52(4):415-20

Sunderland T: Differential cholinergic regulation in Alzheimer's patients compared to controls following chronic blockade with scopolamine: - a SPECT study. Psychopharmacology (Berl) 1995 Sep;121(2):231-41

Talbot PR. A clinical role for 99mTc-HMPAO SPECT in the investigation of dementia? J Neurol Neurosurg Psychiatry 1998 Mar;64(3):306-13

Tanaka S. Inferior temporal lobe atrophy and APOE genotypes in Alzheimer's disease. X-ray computed tomography, magnetic resonance imaging and Xe-133 SPECT studies. Dement Geriatr Cogn Disord 1998 Mar-Apr;9(2):90-8

Tsolaki M. Correlation of rCBF (SPECT), CSF tau, and cognitive function in patients with dementia of the Alzheimer's type, other types of dementia, and control subjects. Am J Alzheimers Dis Other Demen 2001 Jan-Feb;16(1):21-31

Valladares-Neto DC. EEG delta, positron emission tomography, and memory deficit in Alzheimer's disease. Neuropsychobiology 1995;31(4):173-81

van Dyck CH. Comparison of technetium-99m-HMPAO and technetium-99m-ECD cerebral SPECT images in Alzheimer's disease. J Nucl Med 1996 Nov;37(11):1749-55

van Dyck CH. Absence of an apolipoprotein E epsilon4 allele is associated with increased parietal regional cerebral blood flow asymmetry in Alzheimer disease. Arch Neurol 1998 Nov;55(11):1460-6

Van Gool WA. Diagnosing Alzheimer's disease in elderly, mildly demented patients: the impact of routine single photon emission computed tomography. J Neurol 1995 Jun;242(6):401-5

Varrone A. Comparison between cortical distribution of I-123 iomazenil and Tc-99m HMPAO in patients with Alzheimer's disease using SPECT. Clin Nucl Med 1999 Sep;24(9):660-5

Waldemar G: Functional brain imaging with single-photon emission computed tomography in the diagnosis of Alzheimer's disease. Int Psychogeriatr, 9 Suppl 1():223-7; discussion 247-52 1997

Waldemar G. Functional brain imaging with SPECT in normal aging and dementia. Methodological, pathophysiological, and diagnostic aspects. Cerebrovasc Brain Metab Rev 1995 Summer;7(2):89-130

Waldemar G. Heterogeneity of neocortical cerebral blood flow deficits in dementia of the Alzheimer type: a [99mTc]-d,l-HMPAO SPECT study. J Neurol Neurosurg Psychiatry 1994 Mar;57(3):285-95.

Woods SW: SPECT regional cerebral blood flow and neuropsychological testing in non-demented HIV-positive drug abusers: preliminary results. Prog Neuropsychopharmacol Biol Psychiatry 1991;15(5):649-62

Wszolek ZK: Comparison of EEG background frequency analysis, psychologic test scores, short test of mental status, and quantitative SPECT in dementia. J Geriatr Psychiatry Neurol 1992 Jan-Mar;5(1):22-30

Wolfe N. Temporal lobe perfusion on single photon emission computed tomography predicts the rate of cognitive decline in Alzheimer's disease. Arch Neurol 1995 Mar;52(3):257-62

Wyper D. Abnormalities in rCBF and computed tomography in patients with Alzheimer's disease and in controls. Br J Radiol 1993 Jan;66(781):23-7

Zimmer R. Variability of cerebral blood flow deficits in 99mTc-HMPAO SPECT in patients with Alzheimer's disease. J Neural Transm 1997;104(6-7):689-701

Depression/Affective Disorders

Austin MP: Single photon emission tomography with 99mTc-exametazime in major depression and the pattern of brain activity underlying the psychotic/neurotic continuum. J Affect Disord 1992 Sep;26(1):31-43

Bench CJ: The anatomy of melancholia—focal abnormalities of cerebral blood flow in major depression. Psychol Med 1992 Aug;22(3):607-15

Bonne O: Increased cerebral blood flow in depressed patients responding to electroconvulsive therapy. J Nucl Med, 37(7):1075-80 1996 Jul

Bromfield EB. Cerebral metabolism and depression in patients with complex partial seizures. Arch Neurol 1992 Jun;49(6):617-23.

Cummings JL. The neuroanatomy of depression. J Clin Psychiatry 1993 Nov;54:14-20.

Curran SM. A single photon emission computerised tomography study of regional brain function in elderly patients with major depression and with Alzheimer-type dementia. Br J Psychiatry 1993 Aug;163():155-65.

Dolan RJ: Neuropsychological dysfunction in depression: the relationship to regional cerebral blood flow. Psychol Med 1994 Nov;24(4):849-57

Ebert D. A test-retest study of cerebral blood flow during somatosensory stimulation in depressed patients with schizophrenia and major depression. Eur Arch Psychiatry Clin Neurosci 1993;242(4):250-4.

Folk S. Evaluation of the effects of total sleep deprivation on cerebral blood flow using single photon emission computerized tomography. Acta Psychiatr Scand 1992 Dec;86(6):478-83.

Galynker: Hypofrontality and negative symptoms in major depressive disorder. J Nucl Med, 39(4):608-12 1998 Apr

George MS: Brain activity during transient sadness and happiness in healthy women. Am J Psychiatry 1995 Mar;152(3):341-51

George MS. SPECT and PET imaging in mood disorders. J Clin Psychiatry 1993 Nov;54 Suppl():6-13.

Hornig M: HMPAO SPECT brain imaging in treatment-resistant depression. Prog Neuropsychopharmacol Biol Psychiatry, 21(7):1097-114 1997 Oct

Kanaya T. Regional cerebral blood flow in depression. Jpn J Psychiatry Neurol 1990 Sep;44(3):571-6.

Kawakatsu S: Xe-133 inhalation single photon emission computerized tomography in manic-depressive illness. Nippon Rinsho 1994 May;52(5):1180-4

Mayberg HS. Paralimbic hypoperfusion in unipolar depression. J Nucl Med 1994 Jun;35(6):929-34.

Nobler MS: Regional cerebral blood flow in mood disorders, III. Treatment and clinical response. Arch Gen Psychiatry 1994 Nov;51(11):884-97

O'Connell RA. Single-photon emission computed tomography of the brain in acute mania and schizophrenia. J Neuroimaging 1995 Apr;5(2):101-4.

Philpot MP. 99mTc-HMPAO single photon emission tomography in late life depression: a pilot study of regional cerebral blood flow at rest and during a verbal fluency task. J Affect Disord 1993 Aug;28(4):233-40.

Sackeim HA. Regional cerebral blood flow in mood disorders. I. Comparison of major depressives and normal controls at rest. Arch Gen Psychiatry 1990 Jan;47(1):60-70

Sackeim HA. Regional cerebral blood flow in mood disorders. II. Comparison of major depression and Alzheimer's disease. J Nucl Med 1993 Jul;34(7):1090-101.

Schneider F. Differential effects of mood on cortical cerebral blood flow: a 133xenon clearance study. Psychiatry Res 1994 May;52(2):215-36.

Schwartz RB. SPECT imaging of the brain: comparison of findings in patients with chronic fatigue syndrome, AIDS dementia complex, and major unipolar depression. AJR Am J Roentgenol 1994 Apr;162(4):943-51.

Scott AI: Short-term effects of electroconvulsive treatment on the uptake of 99mTc-exametazime into brain in major depression shown with single photon emission tomography. J Affect Disord 1994 Jan;30(1):27-34

Soares JC: The functional neuroanatomy of mood disorders. Psychiatr Res, 31(4):393-432 1997 Jul-Aug

Thomas P. Cerebral blood flow in major depression and dysthymia. J Affect Disord 1993 Dec;29(4):235-42.

Eating Disorders

Krieg JC: Brain morphology and regional cerebral blood flow in anorexia nervosa. Biol Psychiatry 1989 Apr 15;25(8):1041-8

Kuruoglu AC: Tc-99m-HMPAO brain SPECT in anorexia nervosa. J Nucl Med, 39(2):304-6 1998 Feb

Nozoe S: Comparison of regional cerebral blood flow in patients with eating disorders. Brain Res Bull 1995;36(3):251-5

Nozoe S. Changes in regional cerebral blood flow in patients with anorexia nervosa detected through single photon emission tomography imaging. Biol Psychiatry 1993 Oct 15;34(8):578-80.

Gilles de la Tourette's Disorder

George MS, Trimble MR. Elevated frontal cerebral blood flow in Gilles de la Tourette syndrome: a 99Tcm-HMPAO SPECT study. Psychiatry Res 1992 Nov;45(3):143-51.

Lampreave JL: Technetium-99m-HMPAO in Tourette's syndrome on neuroleptic therapy and after withdrawal. J Nucl Med, 39(4):624-8 1998 Apr

Moriarty J: Brain perfusion abnormalities in Gilles de la Tourette's syndrome. Br J Psychiatry 1995 Aug; 167(2):249-54

Steven S: Tourette Syndrome: Prediction of Phenotypic Variation in Monozygotic Twins by Caudate Nucleus D2 Receptor Binding. SCIENCE, Vol. 273, 30 August 1996, pg. 1225

Headache

Bes A, Fabre N: Cerebral blood flow in migraine without aura. REVIEW ARTICLE: 38 REFS. Pathol Biol (Paris) 1992 Apr;40(4):325-31

Gilkey SJ: Cerebral blood flow in chronic posttraumatic headache. Headache, 37(9):583-7 1997 Oct

Soriani S: Interictal and ictal phase study with Tc 99m HMPAO brain SPECT in juvenile migraine with aura. Headache, 37(1):31-6 1997 Jan

Trucco M: Piroxicam-beta-cyclodextrin in induced migraine attacks: a SPECT study with Tc-99m HM-PAO split-dose method. Funct Neurol 1994 Sep-Oct;9(5):247-57

Uhlig B, Stefan H: Functional and structural follow-up findings in complicated migraine. Nervenarzt 1993 Feb;64(2):127-30

Brain Infections

Kao CH:Tc-99m HMPAO brain SPECT findings in pediatric viral encephalitis. Clin Nucl Med, 19(7):590-4 1994 Jul

Launes J: Unilateral hyperfusion in brain-perfusion SPECT predicts poor prognosis in acute encephalitis. Neurology, 48(5):1347-51 1997 May

Medication and Other Treatment Effects

Agnoli A: CBF and cognitive evaluation of Alzheimer type patients before and after IMAO-B treatment: a pilot study. Eur Neuropsychopharmacol 1992 Mar;2(1):31-5

Ebmeier KP: Effects of a single dose of the acetylcholinesterase inhibitor velnacrine on recognition memory and regional cerebral blood flow in Alzheimer's disease. Psychopharmacology (Berl) 1992;108(1-2):103-9

Friston KJ: Measuring the neuromodulatory effects of drugs in man with positron emission tomography. Neurosci Lett 1992 Jul 6;141(1):106-10

Hoehn-Saric R: Effects of fluoxetine on regional cerebral blood flow in obsessive-compulsive patients. Am J Psychiatry 1991 Sep;148(9):1243-5

Hoehn-Saric R: A fluoxetine-induced frontal lobe syndrome in an obsessive compulsive patient. J Clin Psychiatry 1991 Mar;52(3):131-3

Jibiki I: Acutely administered haloperidol-induced pattern changes of regional cerebral blood flow in schizophrenics. Observation from subtraction of brain imaging with single photon emission computed tomography using technetium-99m hexamethyl-propyleneamine oxime. Neuropsychobiology 1992;25(4):182-7

Laatsch L: Impact of cognitive rehabilitation therapy on neuropsychological impairments as measured by brain perfusion SPECT: a longitudinal study. Brain Inj, 11(12):851-63 1997 Dec

McMackin D: Regional cerebral blood flow and language dominance: SPECT during intracarotid amobarbital test.: Neurology, 50(4):943-50 1998 Apr

Mathew RJ: Evaluation of the effects of diazepam and an experimental anti-anxiety drug on regional cerebral blood flow. Psychiatry Res 1991 Oct;40(2):125-34

Miller DD: Effect of antipsychotics on regional cerebral blood flow measured with positron emission tomography. Neuropsychopharmacology, 17(4):230-40 1997 Oct

van Dyck CH: SPECT regional cerebral blood flow alterations in naltrexone-precipitated withdrawal from buprenorphine. Psychiatry Res 1994 Dec;55(4):181-91

Vasile RG: Changes in regional cerebral blood flow following light treatment for seasonal affective disorder: responders versus nonresponders. Biol Psychiatry, 42(11):1000-5 1997 Dec 1

Watanabe MD: Successful methylphenidate treatment of apathy after subcortical infarcts. J Neuropsychiatry Clin Neurosci 1995 Fall;7(4):502-4

Memory Loss/Cognitive Impairment/Dyslexia

Araki S: Reading and writing deficit in cases of localized infarction of the left anterior thalamus. To Shinkei 1990 Jan;42(1):65-7nn2

Attig E, Botez MI: Cerebral crossed diaschisis caused by cerebellar lesion: role of the cerebellum in mental functions. Av Neurol (Paris) 1991;147(3):200-.

Boivin MJ: Verbal fluency and positron emission tomographic mapping of regional cerebral glucose metabolism. Cortex 1992 Jun;28(2):231-9

Evans J: Neuropsychological and SPECT scan findings during and after transient global amnesia: evidence for the differential impairment of remote episodic memory. J Neurol Neurosurg Psychiatry 1993 Nov;56(11):1227-30

Flowers DL: Regional cerebral blood flow correlates of language processes in reading disability. Arch Neurol 1991 Jun;48(6):637-43

Hanyu H: 123I-IMP SPECT study on patients with amnestic syndrome. Kaku Igaku 1992 Jun;29(6):691-4

Hokkanen L: Isolated retrograde amnesia for autobiographical material associated with acute left temporal lobe encephalitis. Psychol Med 1995 Jan;25(1):203-8

Horwitz B: Functional connectivity of the angular gyrus in normal reading and dyslexia. Proc Natl Acad Sci U S A, 95(15):8939-44 1998 Jul

Jibiki I: Case study of monosymptomatic delusion of unpleasant body odor with structural frontal abnormality. Neuropsychobiology 1994;30(1):7-10

Kim MH: Amnesia syndrome following left anterior thalamic infarction; with intrahemispheric and crossed cerebro-cerebellar diaschisis on brain SPECT. J Korean Med Sci 1994 Oct;9(5):427-31

Ohnishi T: High-resolution SPECT to assess hippocampal perfusion in neuropsychiatric diseases. J Nucl Med 1995 Jul;36(7):1163-9

Obsessive Compulsive Disorder/Spectrum

Adams BL: Single photon emission computerized tomography in obsessive compulsive disorder: a preliminary study. J Psychiatry Neurosci 1993 May;18(3):109-12

Baxter LR Jr: Neuroimaging studies of obsessive compulsive disorder. Psychiatr Clin North Am 1992 Dec;15(4):871-84

Baxter LR Jr: Positron emission tomography studies of cerebral glucose metabolism in obsessive compulsive disorder. J Clin Psychiatry 1994 Oct;55 Suppl:54-9

Biver F: Changes in metabolism of cerebral glucose after stereotactic leukotomy for refractory obsessive-compulsive disorder: a case report. J Neurol Neurosurg Psychiatry 1995 Apr;58(4):502-5

Edmonstone Y: Uptake of 99mTc-exametazime shown by single photon emission computerized tomography in obsessive-compulsive disorder compared with major depression and normal controls. Acta Psychiatr Scand 1994 Oct;90(4):298-303

Flor-Henry P: The obsessive-compulsive syndrome: reflection of fronto-caudate dysregulation of the left hemisphere? Encephale 1990 Jul-Aug;16 Spec No:325-9

Hoehn-Saric R: Effects of fluoxetine on regional cerebral blood flow in obsessive-compulsive patients. Am J Psychiatry 1991 Sep;148(9):1243-5

Hoehn-Saric R: A fluoxetine-induced frontal lobe syndrome in an obsessive compulsive patient. J Clin Psychiatry 1991 Mar;52(3):131-3

Insel TR: Toward a neuroanatomy of obsessive-compulsive disorder. Arch Gen Psychiatry 1992 Sep;49(9):739-44

Laplane D: Obsessive-compulsive and other behavioural changes with bilateral basal ganglia lesions. A magnetic resonance imaging and positron tomography study. Brain 1989 Jun;112 (Pt 3):699-725

Machlin SR: Elevated medial-frontal cerebral blood flow in obsessive-compulsive patients: a SPECT study. Am J Psychiatry 1991 Sep;148(9):1240-2

McGuire PK. Functional anatomy of obsessive-compulsive phenomena. Br J Psychiatry 1994 Apr;164(4):459-68.

Perani D: [18F]FDG PET study in obsessive-compulsive disorder. A clinical/metabolic correlation study after treatment. Br J Psychiatry 1995 Feb;166(2):244-50

Rubin RT: Regional xenon 133 cerebral blood flow and cerebral technetium 99m HMPAO uptake in unmedicated patients with obsessive-compulsive disorder and matched normal control subjects. Determination by high-resolution single-photon emission computed tomography. Arch Gen Psychiatry 1992 Sep;49(9):695-702

Sawle GV: Obsessional slowness. Functional studies with positron emission tomography. Brain 1991 Oct;114 (Pt 5):2191-202

Simpson S. Neuropsychiatry and SPECT of an acute obsessive-compulsive syndrome patient. Br J Psychiatry 1995 Mar;166(3):390-2.

Schizophrenia

Blackwood DH. Correlation of regional cerebral blood flow equivalents measured by single photon emission computerized tomography with P300 latency and eye movement abnormality in schizophrenia. Acta Psychiatr Scand 1994 Sep;90(3):157-66.

Busatto GF. Regional cerebral blood flow (rCBF) in schizophrenia during verbal memory activation: a 99mTc-HMPAO single photon emission tomography (SPET) study. Psychol Med 1994 May;24(2):463-72.

Ceballos C: Chronic schizophrenia: validity of the study of regional cerebral blood flow through cerebral SPECT. Rev Neurol, 25(145):1346-9 1997 Sep

Ceballos C: Reliability of the evaluation of regional cerebral blood flow using SPECT in chronic schizophrenia and bipolar disorder. Actas Luso Esp Neurol Psiquiatr Cienc Afines, 26(1):35-40 1998 Jan-Feb

Gordon E: Single photon emission computed tomography (SPECT) measures of brain function in schizophrenia. Aust N Z J Psychiatry 1994 Sep;28(3):446-52

Gunther W: MRI-SPECT and PET-EEG findings on brain dysfunction in schizophrenia. Prog Neuropsychopharmacol Biol Psychiatry 1992 Jul;16(4):445-62

Gunther W. Brain dysfunction during motor activation and corpus callosum alterations in schizophrenia measured by cerebral blood flow and magnetic resonance imaging. Biol Psychiatry 1991 Mar 15;29(6):535-55.

Kawasaki Y. Regional cerebral blood flow in patients with schizophrenia. A preliminary report. Eur Arch Psychiatry Clin Neurosci 1992;241(4):195-200.

Kawasaki Y. SPECT analysis of regional cerebral blood flow changes in patients with schizophrenia during the Wisconsin Card Sorting Test. Schizophr Res 1993 Aug;10(2):109-16.

Matsui M: Saccadic eye movements and regional cerebral blood flow in schizophrenic patients. Eur Arch Psychiatry Clin Neurosci, 247(4):219-27 1997

Musalek M. Regional brain function in hallucinations: a study of regional cerebral blood flow with 99m-Tc-HMPAO-SPECT in patients with auditory hallucinations, tactile hallucinations, and normal controls. Compr Psychiatry 1989 Jan-Feb;30(1):99-108.

Rubin P. Relationship between brain structure and function in disorders of the schizophrenic spectrum: single positron emission computerized tomography, computerized tomography and psychopathology of first episodes. Acta Psychiatr Scand 1994 Oct;90(4):281-9.

Rubin P. Regional cerebral blood flow distribution in newly diagnosed schizophrenia and schizophreniform disorder. Psychiatry Res 1994 Jul;53(1):57-75.

Sagawa K: Correlation of regional cerebral blood flow with performance on neuro-psychological tests in schizophrenic patients. Schizophr Res 1990 Jul-Aug;3(4):241-6

Satoh K. Functional brain imaging of a catatonic type of schizophrenia: PET and SPECT studies. J Psychiatry Neurol 1993 Dec;47(4):881-5.

Sieg KG: Brain imaging: evoked potential, quantitative EEG and SPECT abnormalities in schizophrenia. J Psychiatry Neurosci 1991 Mar;16(1):41-4

Volz HP: Brain activation during cognitive stimulation with the Wisconsin Card Sorting Test—a functional MRI study on healthy volunteers and schizophrenics. Psychiatry Res, 75(3):145-57 1997 Oct 31

Seizures/Partial Seizures

Adamsbaum C. Accelerated myelination in early Sturge-Weber syndrome: MRI-SPECT correlations. Pediatr Radiol 1996 Nov;26(11):759-62

Aguilar Rebolledo F. SPECT-99mTc-HMPAO in a case of epilepsia partialis continua and focal encephalitis. [Article in Spanish] Rev Invest Clin 1996 May-Jun;48(3):199-205

Alper E. Tc-99m HMPAO brain SPECT compared to CT and EEG after seizures in childhood. Clin Nucl Med 1995 Sep;20(9):803-6

Arnold S. Ictal SPECT hyperperfusion reflects the activation of the symptomatogenic cortex in spontaneous and electrically-induced non-habitual focal epileptic seizures: correlation with subdural EEG recordings. Epileptic Disord 2000 Mar;2(1):41-4

Avery RA. Decreased cerebral blood flow during seizures with ictal SPECT injections. Epilepsy Res 2000 Jun;40(1):53-61

Avery RA. Reproducibility of serial peri-ictal single-photon emission tomography difference images in epilepsy patients undergoing surgical resection. Eur J Nucl Med 2000 Jan;27(1):50-5

Aylett SE. Sturge-Weber syndrome: cerebral haemodynamics during seizure activity. Dev Med Child Neurol 1999 Jul;41(7):480-5

Baumgartner C. Regional cerebral blood flow during temporal lobe seizures associated with ictal vomiting: an ictal SPECT study in two patients. Epilepsia 1999 Aug;40(8):1085-91

Baumgartner C: Preictal SPECT in temporal lobe epilepsy: regional cerebral blood flow is increased prior to electroencephalography-seizure onset. J Nucl Med, 39(6):978-82 1998 Jun

Biraben A. Video-EEG and ictal SPECT in three patients with both epileptic and non-epileptic seizures. Epileptic Disord 1999 Mar;1(1):51-5

Biraben A. Fear as the main feature of epileptic seizures. J Neurol Neurosurg Psychiatry 2001 Feb;70(2):186-91

Blend MJ. Cerebral perfusion SPECT imaging in epileptic and nonepileptic seizures. Clin Nucl Med 1997 Jun;22(6):363-8

Bohnen NI. Cerebellar changes in partial seizures: clinical correlations of quantitative SPECT and MRI analysis. Epilepsia 1998 Jun;39(6):640-50

Børch K: Regional cerebral blood flow during seizures in neonates. J Pediatr, 132(3 Pt 1):431-5 1998 Mar

Boussion N. Towards an optimal reference region in single-photon emission tomography difference images in epilepsy. Eur J Nucl Med 2000 Feb;27(2):155-60

Brinkmann BH. Subtraction ictal SPECT coregistered to MRI for seizure focus localization in partial epilepsy. Mayo Clin Proc 2000 Jun;75(6):615-24

Brinkmann BH. Dual-isotope SPECT using simultaneous acquisition of 99mTc and 123I radioisotopes: a double-injection technique for peri-ictal functional neuroimaging. J Nucl Med 1999 Apr;40(4):677-84

Bulakhova LA. Cerebral blood flow in children and adolescents with epilepsy. Zh Nevropatol Psikhiatr Im S S Korsakova 1986;86(6):805-10

Chiron C: A serial study of regional cerebral blood flow before and after hemispherectomy in a child. Epilepsy Res 1991 Apr;8(3):232-40

Chiron C. Study of the cerebral blood flow in partial epilepsy of childhood using the SPECT method. J Neuroradiol 1989 Dec;16(4):317-24

Chiron C. Brain functional imaging SPECT in agyria-pachygyria. Epilepsy Res 1996 Jun;24(2):109-17

Cross JH. Children with intractable focal epilepsy: ictal and interictal 99TcM HMPAO single photon emission computed tomography. Dev Med Child Neurol 1995 Aug;37(8):673-81

Cross JH. Interictal 99Tc(m) HMPAO SPECT and 1H MRS in children with temporal lobe epilepsy. Epilepsia 1997 Mar;38(3):338-45

Dasheiff RM. A review of interictal cerebral blood flow in the evaluation of patients for epilepsy surgery. Seizure 1992 Jun;1(2):117-25

d'Asseler YM. Recent and future evolutions in NeuroSPECT with particular emphasis on the synergistic use and fusion of imaging modalities. Acta Neurol Belg 1997 Sep;97(3):154-62

Denays R, Rubinstein M, Ham H, Piepsz A, Noel P: Single photon emission computed tomography in seizure disorders. Arch Dis Child 1988 Oct;63(10):1184-8

Devous MD Sr: SPECT brain imaging in epilepsy: a meta-analysis. J Nucl Med, 39(2):285-93 1998 Feb

Dierckx RA. Single photon emission computed tomography using perfusion tracers in seizure disorders. Epilepsy Res 1992 Jul;12(2):131-9

Dietrich ME: Correlation of abnormalities of interictal n-isopropyl-p-iodoamphetamine single-photon emission tomography with focus of seizure onset in complex partial seizure disorders. Epilepsia 1991 Mar-Apr;32(2):187-94

Dominguez-Gadea L. Cerebral perfusion during word repetition in epileptic patients. Rev Neurol 2001 Jan 1-15;32(1):6-10

Dressler D: The development of an epileptogenic focus. A case study with 99mTc-HMPAO SPECT. J Neurol 1989 Jul;236(5):300-2

Duncan JS. Imaging and epilepsy. Brain 1997 Feb;120 (Pt 2):339-77

Duncan R. Ictal/postictal SPECT in the pre-surgical localisation of complex partial seizures. J Neurol Neurosurg Psychiatry 1993 Feb;56(2):141-8.

Duncan R: Ictal regional cerebral blood flow in frontal lobe seizures. Seizure, 6(5):393-401 1997 Oct

Duncan R. Ictal single photon emission computed tomography in occipital lobe seizures. Epilepsia 1997 Jul;38(7):839-43

Duncan JD. Use of positron emission tomography for presurgical localization of eloquent brain areas in children with seizures. Pediatr Neurosurg 1997 Mar;26(3):144-56

Duncan R. Ictal cerebral blood flow in seizures originating in the posterolateral cortex. J Nucl Med 1996 Dec;37(12):1946-51

Duncan R. Interictal temporal hypoperfusion is related to early-onset temporal lobe epilepsy. Epilepsia 1996 Feb;37(2):134-40

Duncan R. Tc99m HM-PAO single photon emission computed tomography in temporal lobe epilepsy. Acta Neurol Scand 1990 Apr;81(4):287-93

English R: Five patients with Rasmussen's syndrome investigated by single-photon-emission computed tomography. Nucl Med Commun 1989 Jan;10(1):5-14

Flamini JR: I-123 SPECT scan in children with neurological disorders. Wis Med J 1990 Oct;89(10):584-7

Griffiths PD. 99mTechnetium HMPAO imaging in children with the Sturge-Weber syndrome: a study of nine cases with CT and MRI correlation. Neuroradiology 1997 Mar; 39(3):219-24

Grunwald F: Technetium-99m-HMPAO brain SPECT in medically intractable, temporal lobe epilepsy: a postoperative evaluation. J Nucl Med 1991 Mar;32(3):388-94

Grunwald F. Single-photon, emission-computed tomography (SPECT) in the diagnosis of epilepsy. Radiologe 1993 Apr;33(4):198-203

Grunwald F. HMPAO-SPECT in cerebral seizures. Nuklearmedizin 1988 Dec;27(6):248-51

Guerreiro MM. Brain single photon emission computed tomography imaging in Landau-Kleffner syndrome. Epilepsia 1996 Jan;37(1):60-7

Guillon B: Correlation between interictal regional cerebral blood flow and depth-recorded interictal spiking in temporal lobe epilepsy. Epilepsia, 39(1):67-76 1998 Jan

Gulati S. Single-photon emission computed tomography (SPECT) in childhood epilepsy. Indian J Pediatr 2000 Jan;67(1 Suppl):S32-9

Hara M: Single photon emission computed tomography in children with idiopathic seizures. Radiat Med 1991 Sep-Oct;9(5):185-9

Haginoya K. The perfusion defect seen with SPECT in West syndrome is not correlated with seizure prognosis or developmental outcome. Brain Dev 2000 Jan;22(1):16-23

Hara M: 123I-IMP single photon emission computed tomography (SPECT) study in childhood epilepsy. Kaku Igaku 1990 Nov;27(11):1239-45

Harvey AS. Functional neuroimaging with SPECT in children with partial epilepsy. J Child Neurol 1994 Oct;9 Suppl 1:S71-81.

Harvey AS. Frontal lobe epilepsy: clinical seizure characteristics and localization with ictal 99mTc-HMPAO SPECT. Neurology 1993 Oct;43(10):1966-80

Heiskala H. Brain perfusion SPECT in children with frequent fits. Brain Dev 1993 May-Jun;15(3):214-8

Henkes H: Increased rCBF in gray matter heterotopias detected by SPECT using 99mTc hexamethyl-propylenamine oxime. Neuroradiology 1991;33(4):310-2

Henry TR. Acute blood flow changes and efficacy of vagus nerve stimulation in partial epilepsy. Neurology 1999 Apr 12;52(6):1166-73

Henry TR. Brain blood flow alterations induced by therapeutic vagus nerve stimulation in partial epilepsy: I. Acute effects at high and low levels of stimulation. Epilepsia 1998 Sep;39(9):983-90

Ho SS. Temporal lobe epilepsy subtypes: differential patterns of cerebral perfusion on ictal SPECT. Epilepsia 1996 Aug;37(8):788-95

Hollo A. Ictal perfusion changes during occipital lobe seizures in infancy: report of two serial ictal observations. Epilepsia 2001 Feb;42(2):275-9

Homan RW: Cognitive function and regional cerebral blood flow in partial seizures. Arch Neurol 1989 Sep;46(9):964-70

Hwang SI. Comparative analysis of MR imaging, positron emission tomography, and ictal single-photon emission CT in patients with neocortical epilepsy. AJNR Am J Neuroradiol 2001 May;22(5):937-46

Hwang PA. Infantile spasms: cerebral blood flow abnormalities correlate with EEG, neuroimaging, and pathologic findings. Pediatr Neurol 1996 Apr;14(3):220-5

Iannetti P. Neuronal migrational disorders in children with epilepsy: MRI, interictal SPECT and EEG comparisons. Brain Dev 1996 Jul-Aug;18(4):269-79

Ide M. A case of temporal lobe epilepsy with improvement of clinical symptoms and single photon emission computed tomography findings after treatment with clonazepam. Psychiatry Clin Neurosci 2000 Oct;54(5):595-7

Janicek MJ. Quantitative evaluation of 99mTc-hexamethylpropylenamineoxime brain SPECT in childhood-onset epilepsy. J Nucl Biol Med 1992 Oct-Dec;36(4):319-23

Jibiki I. Correlations between quantitative EEG and regional cerebral blood flow (SPECT) in patients with partial epilepsy. Neuropsychobiology 1994;30(1):46-52.

Jibiki I: High reproducibility of regional abnormalities on interictal 123I-IMP SPECT brain scans in adults with partial epilepsy. Eur Arch Psychiatry Neurol Sci 1990;240(1):5-8

Jha SK. Interictal brain 99m Tc-HMPAO SPECT study in cases of epilepsy with single ring enhancing CT lesion. J Assoc Physicians India 2000 Apr;48(4):382-5

Jha SK. Interictal brain 99m Tc-HMPAO SPECT study in chronic epilepsy. J Assoc Physicians India 1998 May;46(5):438-41

Kanazawa O: 99mTc-HMPAO SPECT in epileptic disorders in childhood. No To Hattatsu 1991 Nov;23(6):601-5

Kapucu LO. Brain SPECT evaluation of patients with pure photosensitive epilepsy. J Nucl Med 1996 Nov;37(11):1755-9

Karagol U. Cerebral blood flow abnormalities in symptomatic West syndrome: a single photon emission computed tomography study. Pediatr Int 2001 Feb;43(1):66-70

Katayama S, Momose T, Sano I, Nakashima Y, Nakajima T, Niwa S, Matsushita M. The mechanism of controlling regional cerebral blood flow in patients with localization-related epilepsy. Seishin Shinkeigaku Zasshi 1996;98(2):89-114

Kawamura M, Murase K, Kimura H, Hatakeyama T, Mogami H, Kataoka M, Itoh H, Ishine M, Iio A, Hamamoto K, et al: TI - Single photon emission computed tomography (SPECT) using N-isopropyl-p-(123I) iodoamphetamine (IMP) in the evaluation of patients with epileptic seizures. Eur J Nucl Med 1990;16(4-6):285-92

Kawamura M: SPECT with N-isopropyl-p-(123I) iodoamphetamine in partial epilepsy—evaluation of delayed image. Nippon Igaku Hoshasen Gakkai Zasshi 1989 May 25;49(5):630-42

Kawamura M: Visualization of epileptic lesions using single photon emission computed tomography (SPECT) with N-isopropyl-p-(123I) iodoamphetamine after intravenous loading of bemegride—report of a case.

Kim BG. Interpretation of Wada memory test for lateralization of seizure focus by use of (99m)technetium-HMPAO SPECT. Epilepsia 2000 Jan;41(1):65-70

Kim BG. Evaluation of functional changes in the medial temporal region during intracarotid amobarbital procedure by use of SPECT. Epilepsia 1999 Apr;40(4):424-9

Ko D. Vagus nerve stimulation activates central nervous system structures in epileptic patients during PET H2(15)O blood flow imaging. Neurosurgery 1996 Aug;39(2):426-30

Koh S. The localizing value of ictal SPECT in children with tuberous sclerosis complex and refractory partial epilepsy. Epileptic Disord 1999 Mar;1(1):41-6

Konkol RJ: Hemimegalencephaly: clinical, EEG, neuroimaging, and IMP-SPECT correlation. Department of Neurology, Medical College of Wisconsin, Milwaukee. Pediatr Neurol 1990 Nov-Dec;6(6):414-8

LaManna MM: Initial experience with SPECT imaging of the brain using I-123 p-iodoamphetamine in focal epilepsy. Clin Nucl Med 1989 Jun;14(6):428-30

Lancman ME. Usefulness of ictal and interictal 99mTc ethyl cysteinate dimer single photon emission computed tomography in patients with refractory partial epilepsy. Epilepsia 1997 Apr;38(4):466-71

Lang W: Single photon emission computerized tomography during and between seizures. J Neurol 1988 May;235(5):277-84

Launes J. Interictal brain 99Tc-HM-PAO SPECT hypoperfusion in patients with unstable partial epilepsy and normal CT. Acta Neurol Scand 1992 Dec;86(6):558-62

Lawson JA. Evaluation of SPECT in the assessment and treatment of intractable childhood epilepsy. Neurology 2000 Nov 14;55(9):1391-3

Lee DS. Late postictal residual perfusion abnormality in epileptogenic zone found on 6-hour postictal SPECT. Neurology 2000 Sep 26;55(6):835-41

Lee HW, Hong SB, Tae WS. Opposite ictal perfusion patterns of subtracted SPECT. Hyperperfusion and hypoperfusion. Brain 2000 Oct;123 (Pt 10):2150-9

Lee SK. The clinical usefulness of ictal SPECT in temporal lobe epilepsy: the lateralization of seizure focus and correlation with EEG. Epilepsia 2000 Aug;41(8):955-62

Lemesle M. Correlation between inter-ictal regional cerebral blood flow and sphenoidal electrodes—recorded inter-ictal spikes in mesial temporal lobe epilepsy. Neurol Res 2000 Oct;22(7):674-8

Lynch BJ. Correlation of 99mTc-HMPAO SPECT with EEG monitoring: prognostic value for outcome of epilepsy surgery in children. Brain Dev 1995 Nov-Dec;17(6):409-417

Maehara T. Interictal hyperperfusion observed in infants with cortical dysgenesis. Brain Dev 1999 Sep;21(6):407-12

Markand ON. Comparative study of interictal PET and ictal SPECT in complex partial seizures. Acta Neurol Scand 1997 Mar;95(3):129-36

Marks DA. Localization of extratemporal epileptic foci during ictal single photon emission computed tomography. Ann Neurol 1992 Mar;31(3):250-5

Marrosu F. Correlation between cerebral perfusion and hyperventilation enhanced focal spiking activity. Epilepsy Res 2000 Jun;40(1):79-86

Mastin ST. Prospective localization of epileptogenic foci: comparison of PET and SPECT with site of surgery and clinical outcome. Radiology 1996 May;199(2):375-80

Matsuda H. Interictal cerebral and cerebellar blood flow in temporal lobe epilepsy as measured by a noninvasive technique using Tc-99m HMPAO. Clin Nucl Med 1996 Nov;21(11):867-72

Menzel C. Brain single-photon emission tomography using technetium-99m bicisate (ECD) in a case of complex partial seizure. Eur J Nucl Med 1994 Nov;21(11):1243-6

Menzel C. Evaluation of technetium-99m-ECD in childhood epilepsy. J Nucl Med 1996 Jul;37(7):1106-12

Noachtar S. Ictal technetium-99m ethyl cysteinate dimer single-photon emission tomographic findings and propagation of epileptic seizure activity in patients with extratemporal epilepsies. Eur J Nucl Med 1998 Feb;25(2):166-72

O'Brien TJ. Subtraction peri-ictal SPECT is predictive of extratemporal epilepsy surgery outcome. Neurology 2000 Dec 12;55(11):1668-77

O'Brien TJ. The practical utility of performing peri-ictal SPECT in the evaluation of children with partial epilepsy. Pediatr Neurol 1998 Jul;19(1):15-22

Okuchi K. Regional cerebral blood flow after status epilepticus. Keio J Med 2000 Feb;49 Suppl 1:A75-6

Oliveira AJ. Localization of the epileptogenic zone by ictal and interictal SPECT with 99mTc-ethyl cysteinate dimer in patients with medically refractory epilepsy. Epilepsia 1999 Jun;40(6):693-702

Otsubo H. Location of epileptic foci on interictal and immediate postictal single photon emission tomography in children with localization-related epilepsy. J Child Neurol 1995 Sep;10(5):375-81

Otsubo H. Focal cortical dysplasia in children with localization-related epilepsy: EEG, MRI, and SPECT findings. Pediatr Neurol 1993 Mar-Apr;9(2):101-7

Otsubo H: Neuroimaging studies in children with temporal lobectomy. Childs Nerv Syst 1995 May;11(5):281-7

Packard AB. Ictal and interictal technetium-99m-bicisate brain SPECT in children with refractory epilepsy. J Nucl Med 1996 Jul;37(7):1101-6

Perlman JM. Positron emission tomography in the newborn: effect of seizure on regional cerebral blood flow in an asphyxiated infant. Neurology 1985 Feb;35(2):244-7

Podreka I: Hexa-methyl-propylene-amine-oxime (HMPAO) single photon emission computed tomography (SPECT) in epilepsy. Brain Topogr 1988 Fall;1(1):55-60

Rodrigues M. Combined study of 99mTc-HMPAO SPECT and computerized electroencephalographic topography (CET) in patients with medically refractory complex partial epilepsy. Ann Nucl Med 1996 Feb;10(1):113-8

Rougier A. Bilateral decrease in interictal hippocampal blood flow in unilateral mesiotemporal epilepsy. J Neurosurg 1999 Feb;90(2):282-8

Runge U. Ictal and interictal ECD-SPECT for focus localization in epilepsy. Acta Neurol Scand 1997 Nov;96(5):271-6

Sackeim HA. The anticonvulsant hypothesis of the mechanisms of action of ECT: current status. J ECT 1999 Mar;15(1):5-26

San Pedro EC. Anterior cingulate gyrus epilepsy: the role of ictal rCBF SPECT in seizure localization. Epilepsia 2000 May;41(5):594-600

Sarikaya A, Kaya M, Karasalihoglu S, Alemdar A, Altun G, Berkarda S. Comparison between semiquantitative interictal Tc-99m HMPAO SPECT and clinical parameters in children with partial seizures. Brain Dev 1999 Apr;21(3):179-83

Sayit E. Landau-Kleffner syndrome: relation of clinical, EEG and Tc-99m-HMPAO brain SPECT findings and improvement in EEG after treatment. Ann Nucl Med 1999 Dec;13(6):415-8

Sestoft D. Disparity in regional cerebral blood flow during electrically induced seizure. Acta Psychiatr Scand 1993 Aug;88(2):140-3

So EL. Integration of EEG, MRI, and SPECT in localizing the seizure focus for epilepsy surgery. Epilepsia 2000;41 Suppl 3:S48-54

So EL. The EEG evaluation of single photon emission computed tomography abnormalities in epilepsy. J Clin Neurophysiol 2000 Jan;17(1):10-28

Spanaki MV, Spencer SS, Corsi M, MacMullan J, Seibyl J, Zubal IG. The role of quantitative ictal SPECT analysis in the evaluation of nonepileptic seizures. J Neuroimaging 1999 Oct;9(4):210-6

Stefan H. Functional and morphological abnormalities in temporal lobe epilepsy: a comparison of interictal and ictal EEG, CT, MRI, SPECT and PET. J Neurol 1987 Aug;234(6):377-84

Stefan H. Regional cerebral blood flow during focal seizures of temporal and frontocentral onset. Ann Neurol 1990 Feb;27(2):162-6

Studholme C. Estimating tissue deformation between functional images induced by intracranial electrode implantation using anatomical MRI. Neuroimage 2001 Apr;13(4):561-76

Sturm JW. Ictal SPECT and interictal PET in the localization of occipital lobe epilepsy. Epilepsia 2000 Apr;41(4):463-6

Thomas P. Nonconvulsive status epilepticus of frontal origin. Neurology 1999 Apr 12;52(6):1174-83

Uvebrant P: Brain single photon emission computed tomography (SPECT) in neuropediatrics. Neuropediatrics 1991 Feb;22(1):3-9

Van Laere K. Vagus nerve stimulation in refractory epilepsy: SPECT activation study. J Nucl Med 2000 Jul;41(7):1145-54

Van Paesschen W. Self-injection ictal SPECT during partial seizures. Neurology 2000 May 23;54(10):1994-7 \

Vonck K. Acute single photon emission computed tomographic study of vagus nerve stimulation in refractory epilepsy. Epilepsia 2000 May;41(5):601-9

Weinand ME. Temporal lobe seizure interhemispheric propagation time depends on nonepileptic cortical cerebral blood flow. Epilepsy Res 2001 Apr;44(1):33-9

Wichert-Ana L. Typical and atypical perfusion patterns in periictal SPECT of patients with unilateral temporal lobe epilepsy. Epilepsia 2001 May;42(5):660-6

Won HJ. Comparison of MR imaging with PET and ictal SPECT in 118 patients with intractable epilepsy. AJNR Am J Neuroradiol 1999 Apr;20(4):593-9

Won JH. Increased contralateral cerebellar uptake of technetium-99m-HMPAO on ictal brain SPECT. J Nucl Med 1996 Mar;37(3):426-9

Yeni SN. Ictal and interictal SPECT findings in childhood absence epilepsy. Seizure 2000 Jun;9(4):265-9